A Brief Study Course in HOMOEOPATHY

D0839343

by

Elizabeth Wright-Hubbard, M.D.

Fifth Printing 1992
© Formur, Inc., 1977

ISBN 0-89378-071-5

Formur, Inc.—Publishers
4200 Laclede Avenue
St. Louis, MO. 63108

Table of Contents

The Meaning of Homoeopathy. 1
The Epitome of Homoeopathic Philosophy 7
Know the Patient 15
Know the Remedies 23
The Evaluation of the Symptoms. 29
Repertorizing 34
Prescribing: Potency Selection. 44
Repetition 50
Prescribing: Aggravation 55
The Second Prescription 59
Remedy Relationships 61
Pathological Prescribing 66
The Problem of Suppression 69
The Management of the Homoeopathic Patient . .73
Problems Confronting One When First
   Attempting to Prescribe Homoeopathically . . .78
Strange, Rare and Peculiar Symptoms 87
Timing in Prescribing 90
The Value and Relation of Diet
   to our Homoeopathic Remedies 93
The Dangers of Homoeopathic Prescribing 98

We would like to extend our heartfelt appreciation to Mr. Alain Naudé for extending his time and talent to assist us in the preparation of Dr. Elizabeth Wright-Hubbard's manuscript.

THE MEANING OF HOMOEOPATHY

What is Homoeopathy? The orderly mind has a notion one should begin with definition, and resorts first to various dictionaries. In this instance the result is unsatisfactory as the definitions are, for the most part, partial and even the positive statements often inaccurate, as in the case of Dorland's *Medical Dictionary*. As far as derivation goes, the word in the Greek means "similarity of feeling."

The four fundamentals of Homoeopathy, as stated by Hahnemann, in his *Organon,* may be briefly put as follows:

I. The proving of substances to be used as medicines, on the healthy.

II. The selection and administration of so-proved medicines according to the Law of Similars.

III. The single remedy.

IV. The minimum dose.

Granting that these are the four fundamental tenets of Homoeopathy, as set forth by its official sponsor and founder, Hahnemann, the question of the status of Homoeopathy arises. Is it a system of medicine? Is it a purely sectarian term? Is it a therapeutic specialty? In order to be able to answer this question of status we must get down to simple facts, and see not only how Homoeopathy differs from regular medicine but what

1

they have in common. We always like to begin with a common basis. What is the object of all conscientious physicians? We would answer, categorically: To cure the sick, to prevent others from becoming ill, to raise the standard of health in all people. How does modern medicine try to accomplish this? *First,* by finding out what normality is, through the study of anatomy, physiology, physiological chemistry, etc. *Second,* by finding out what the varieties of ill health are. Modern medicine emphasizes the fact that many disturbances of health are due to psychic or sociological causative factors. Aside from these it searches for anatomical or physiological changes in the sick person and classifies these changes, when found, under some disease nomenclature. This search is called diagnosis, and it feels that the possibility of cure depends, in large measure, on the certainty of diagnosis. The organic structural changes due to ill health, which it finds before or after death, it terms pathology. It finds that many "diseases" are accompanied by some variety of bacteria, which it considers to be one of the causative factors. In short, modern medicine feels that it must find out all the "facts" which fit in with its concept of disease.

To all of this the homoeopath subscribes, but he feels that this is but the beginning of what he must learn about his patient. The spontaneous, characteristic things that each patient longs to tell, be they very general or minutely particular, are of special interest to the homoeopath for they individualize the case, bringing out the particular patient's reaction to the "disease" he suffers from. These salient points the busy modern doctor feels that he does not need to know, as to him they are not sign posts but clutter.

At this point modern mecicine is ready to try to cure the disease it has diagnosed. What laws of cure does it follow? First, the common-sense principle of rectifying anything mechanically wrong and instituting appropriate hygiene, diet, etc. When it comes to the giving of actual drugs, each year fewer and fewer are taught in the medical schools and — with the exception of new proprietary substances — are found in the pharmacopoeia or in common usage. Those that are given are not uniformly governed by any one law. The intent is to give them on a physiological basis, which means that they are experimented with in the laboratories in crude dosage, mainly on animals. It is more or less expected, by analogy, that what slows the heart in the frog, rabbit, or dog will do so in the human. Only very occasionally, recently, are pharmacological experiments done on relatively healthy humans. In addition to the laboratory data on animals, many remedies are tried out empirically on patients and pass into general usage in accordance with their success. Some few forms of modern therapy are aimed at the individual as a whole taken as a type, for instance, endocrine therapy, but the majority of modern drugs are given for a definite physiological effect on some one organ or function of the body, and so given irrespective of the varying individualities of the patient, who may have that organ or function disordered, as for instance, cholagogues, digitalis, diuretics, etc., etc. A large part of modern therapy is not even aimed at physiological alteration (the drugs being given according to the law of contraries) nor at chemical antidoting (such as alkalis for acid stomach) but is frankly and only palliative (as in the various anodynes for headaches, neuralgias, etc.). Most of the modern drugging, in short, is aimed at individual annoying symptoms and makes no attempt to get back to the constitutional cause of the disease. The success of this type of therapy is necessarily uneven. More and more modern medicine has come to realize that a great deal of it is suppressive. For instance, some asthma specialists hold that the removal of eczema with salves brings out asthma; some syphilologists hold that the checking of early syphilis by salvarsan and mercury treatment leads to a marked increase in the number of the tertiary neuro-syphilis cases; some medical men feel that heavy salicylate dosage drives rheumatism in on the heart and that the classical quinine does not eradicate malaria, as it often returns yearly or is frequently superseded by neuralgia. It is an interesting fact for further systematic study that many cases of apparent cure prove to be those in which the drug given on a physiological or symptomatic basis was, unknown to the prescriber, a similar, in the homoeopathic sense, to the case in hand.

Let it be, then, clearly understood that homoeopaths need the accepted scientific training, procedures of diagnosis, and laboratory data, that their special technique begins at the moment of starting therapy, although they bring to this crisis of cure a broader philosophy of illness and special knowledge of each individual patient. What this philosophy behind them is, will be the subject of our lecture. What the extra knowledge of the patient must be, and how to get it, will be the subject of a subsequent lecture.

Homoeopathic therapy is based on the hypothesis, ancient as Hippocrates, that like cures likes (*similia similibus curantur*). That this principle is a veridical law of nature, the persistent and enlightened practice of Homoeopathy can prove. It must also be demonstrable by laboratory technique, but the systematic working out of this has not as yet been done, mainly because homoeopaths are so beguiled with the practical application of it that they have not given suitable attention to the laboratory end.

We have sketched modern medicine's approach and attitude and have shown up to what point Homoeopathy concurs. It may not be amiss to give briefly the main points of difference between the two which will be more fully developed in the rest of the course:

1. That there is a natural law of cure, like cures like.

2. That the basis of therapy is a *vital* rather than a *physiological* one, i.e., that the vital force must be stimulated to cure the patient and that only so can he be really cured, that any other drug therapy is palliative or suppressive.

4

3. That the single remedy at a time is all that is needed, which follows from statement 1, because there cannot be two things most similar to another. (The single remedy has the further advantage that when one thing is given one can evaluate its action, whereas, if four are given you cannot know which helped, or in what proportion).

4. That a minimum dose is essential. This is based on the Arndt-Schultz law that small doses stimulate, medium doses paralyze and large doses kill, in other words that the action of small and very large doses of the same substance on living matter is opposite. Under this head comes in the whole potency question of which you will hear more in a later lecture and which is, by many, considered the greatest snag in Homoeopathy but which together with the Law of Similars is the key to the whole matter.

5. That the materia medica must, because of the Law of Similars, be composed of the results of remedy experimentation with small doses on relatively healthy humans (so-called provings).

6. That disease is not an actual entity but a name given for classification purposes to manifestations of departures from normalcy in individuals.

7. That individualization is essential, i.e., that no two people are exactly alike in sickness or in health, and that although even homoeopaths must classify, they draw vastly finer distinctions. For example to ordinary medicine, there is but one disease pneumonia; though with several sub-types, broncho-, lobar, types I, II, III, and IV; to Homoeopathy there are as many types as there are remedy symptom pictures (any drug in the homoeopathic materia medica may be called for in pneumonia although one will rarely need any one outside of thirty or forty in frequent use). Theoretically there should be as many types of pneumonia as there are people who have it, but, owing to the small number of proved remedies compared to the substances that might be proved, there can only be as

5

many pneumonia types to date as we have remedies for. Homoeopaths, in other words classify pneumonias as *Aconite, Bryonia, Gelsemium, Phosphorus, Tartar emetic* pneumonias, etc.

8. That suppression is one of the greatest dangers in medicine. This will be taken up in one of the later lectures.

9. That chronic disease is a constitutional matter and has a philosophic bearing on prescribing, which is of inestimable importance. One cannot do true Homoeopathy without a concept of chronic disease.

Having given the main points of contact and difference between Homoeopathy and regular medicine we can now return to our previous question as to the status of Homoeopathy. It is not a sectarian term, although even a slight study of its history will often show how it has been necessary for it to be considered one, both by its opponents and its adherents. It is a therapeutic specialty and, as such, is more easily grasped by the modern student, but *it is much more than that.* "System of medicine" is a term which conveys little to my mind; it sounds like somebody's textbook or a treatise on one of the minor "opathies." Homoeopathy is not an "opathy," it is the first part of the term, the homoeo, the similarity, which we must bear in mind. It is a method of cure according to law, based, as all great things are, on a far-reaching philosophy. *It is* the central core of medicine, whether recognized or not, and is thoroughly compatible with the best of modern science!

THE EPITOME OF HOMOEOPATHIC PHILOSOPHY

Homoeopathic philosophy may be divided into three sections, the theoretical, dealing with how and why remedies act, which is so abstruse that it can best be dealt with by the more advanced student; the didactic, meaning the rules and tenets; and the practical, which comprises the art of applying the rules in prescribing for the actual patient, understanding the results, and following through the subsequent prescriptions to cure.

First, let us take a bird's eye view of the didactic aspect. Health, to the homoeopath, is a state of harmony between the parts of the body and also between the person as a whole and the cosmos. In real health the as yet unexplained life force in each person is vigorous. It is usually spoken of as the vital force, which in disease is the true curative power. The object of giving the similar remedy is to stimulate the vital force. The object of hygiene and mechanical intervention is to clear its path of obstructions. No remedy can cure disease, it can only at best enable the vital force to function properly again.

Disease, to the homoeopath, is a state of disharmony

involving at least three different factors: some morbific influence, the susceptibility of the person affected, and the individuality of the patient modifying the form the disease takes. Homoeopaths do not try to cure the morbific influence but to cure the patient himself. In order to cure the patient the most similar remedy must be given.

Symptoms, to the homoeopaths, are the language of the body expressing its disharmony and calling for the similar remedy. For prescribing one must take the totality of the symptoms, which includes the mental symptoms; the "generals", predicated of the patient as a whole, which include his reaction to meteorological conditions, time, bodily functions, food, etc.; the particulars, predicated of any part of the patient, and the "modalities" of these (that is, what aggravates or ameliorates), and especially such particulars as are "rare, strange or peculiar"; the causative factors, such as ailments from grief, wetting, riding in a cold wind, suppression of menses, etc.; and the pathological symptoms, indicating the elective affinity of the remedy for certain tissues or organs.

Homoeopathy regards acute disease as an eliminative explosion, which, if handled in the proper homoeopathic manner leaves the body in a healthier condition. This does not mean that the acute disease should be allowed to run its course, for if the symptoms are met at its inception by the *similimum* the disease will be aborted and yet the economy will be purified. No acute case under homoeopathic treatment from the beginning should die, and there should be no permanent sequellae. Acute epidemic diseases often run to one or two epidemic remedies which vary as the disease shifts geographically. In this connection the epidemic remedy is an admirable prophylactic, although the chronic constitutional remedy is always the best preventive. Sequellae following acute diseases are not strictly speaking part of the acute trouble but are flare-ups of chronic disease aroused by the acute condition.

8

Chronic disease is not self-limited and shows no tendency to ultimate recovery if untreated. This is the unique sphere of Homoeopathy. Practically every one has some symptoms of latent chronic disease, and to the homoeopath chronic disease is the basis of susceptibility. By taking the totality of the symptoms from birth on, a deep-acting, chronic constitutional remedy can be chosen which will aid in fending off future acute disease and remove many inherited and acquired encumbrances to the vital force. Hahnemann divided chronic diseases into three main categories or "miasms," psora, syphilis, and sycosis. These may appear singly or in combination with each other or with drug disease engrafted by improper treatment. This matter of the miasms is the most difficult and moot question in Homoeopathy but the fundamental thesis of the importance of chronic disease in general is essential.

Having prescribed for chronic disease, if you have given the true *similimum,* the symptoms are cured in accordance with Hering's three laws of direction: from within outward, from above downward, and in the reverse order of their appearance. This is never the case in chronic disease untreated by Homoeopathy, therefore when observed one can be sure that it is the remedy which is curing and that the correct remedy has been found. Hering's laws are so important that we will give an example: A rheumatic fever case, where the joint symptoms have disappeared and the heart is affected receives the *similimum.* The heart improves, pains return in the shoulders and elbows, these disappear and the knees and ankles are involved, these in turn pass off and the patient entirely recovers. The symptoms went from within outward (heart to joints), from above downward (shoulders to knees), and in the reverse order of their appearance (heart to limbs instead of limbs to heart). If the symptoms do not go in this order the remedy is wrong. When a patient on a chronic remedy develops a different symptom, search back in your record or question your patient rigorously to determine whether this is the recurrence of an old symptom (a good sign, in which case no further remedy should be given). If it is not an old symptom search the pathogenesis of the remedy given. If the symptom appears in the proving give nothing, if not, the choice of the remedy must be revised.

These laws of cure may or may not apply in acute disease, usually they do not. If the picture of a chronic disease includes a suppression, especially if the suppression is due to crude drugging, the chronic remedy acting according to the third law of cure will sometimes restore the original discharge or eruption. The percentage of cases in which this return is from the original channel is relatively low. With good prescribing, however, some exteriorization takes place even though this may only be a diarrhoea or a coryza. One of the times when any practitioner most needs a thorough knowledge of homoeopathic philosophy is when, after chronic prescribing he is faced with such a discharge having more or less acute symptoms. He must then decide whether this is a return of an old trouble in its original form, or a compensatory vent, or a new acute disturbance, or an aggravation. If it is the first he should wait and give *Placebo*, explaining the process to sustain the patient's morale. If it is the second he should attempt to do the same. If, on the other hand it is the third, or the second is too annoying to the patient or even dangerous, one should prescribe an acute remedy and give it in low potency (thirtieth or even the twelfth, surely not above the two hundredth). After this the action of the chronic may not even have been disturbed. Often the acute remedy called for will be found among the acute complements of the chronic remedy. If, in the fourth case, the disturbance is merely an increase in one of the patient's complaints, or is found under the pathogenesis of the chronic remedy given, it can be classed as an aggravation and should receive no medicine, except *Placebo*, unless dangerous as above. If it is so serious as to threaten life, owing to the chronic having been given in too high a potency, an antidote may be in order. The selection of the antidote will be taken up in a later lecture. The great point is not to mix up your case and spoil it by giving unnecessary remedies.

In addition to acute and chronic diseases there are, of course, diseases due to drugging, or to bad hygiene, and there are diseases which have ultimated themselves in pathology calling for surgery, and also troubles which are primarily surgical like foreign bodies, fractures, extra-uterine pregnancy, etc.

A word should be said here about pathology and surgery. From the homoeopathic standpoint much of pathology is protective; abscesses, ulcers, tumors are an effort on the part of the vital force at localization and extrusion. Such pathology should not be removed by surgery until *after* the sick constitution which produced such pathology has been cured. Often in the course of cure the pathology will shrink or be absorbed. If not, it remains as a foreign body and is a subject for surgery. Its removal before the cure of the constitution simply means that, balked at that outlet, the vital force will seek another one, either by recurrence in the same form or by more deep-seated trouble. As to surgery, some of the orthodox homoeopaths hold that any surgery that is not merely a mechanical adjustment (such as ventral suspension of the uterus) is a definite bar to cure, the idea being that in the unraveling of the disease it gets back to where the knot was cut by surgery and can go no further. It requires the keenest judgment to decide when a case has gone too far to be relieved by remedies, and emergency surgery is indicated in a crisis. The homoeopathic remedy should always be resumed after surgery.

In any of these classes of disease where they have been wrongly treated one should include the symptoms of the patient before the incorrect treatment, in other words original symptoms, in the totality.

11

Having glimpsed the didactic aspect we must run over practical philosophy. The unique law which is the basis of all Homoeopathy is *similia similibus curantur*. How we arrive at this equation, the actual studying of drugs and patients is the province of later lectures. The actual handling of cases after the first remedy has been selected is the more difficult part of Homoeopathy. First is the necessity of giving the single remedy. This precludes the use of compound tablets, alternation of remedies, unhomoeopathic adjuvants such as cathartics and anodynes, etc. In a case where the miasms are mixed it may be impossible to cover the totality of the symptoms with one remedy. In such a case observe which miasm is, so to speak, on top and prescribe for the totality of symptoms of *that* miasm, and when these symptoms are cleared off, the layer beneath, representing, perhaps, another miasm, may be prescribed for, again by a single remedy. Sometimes the remedy indicated may be one which has power over all the miasms, as for instance, *Nitric acid*. The single remedy does not mean that only one remedy should be used throughout a case, although that is the desideratum, but simply one remedy at a time. It cannot be too often stated that one must not give a remedy lightly nor change it frequently. In acute diseases the single remedy at a time still holds although the remedy may have to be changed as the case develops, in which case some of our master prescribers hold that the original remedy may be indicated again at the close of the cycle to complete the case. Further details on the single remedy will come up in the lecture on prescribing.

Next in importance to the selection of the single similar remedy is the question of dosage. The classic rule is "the minimum dose." We prefer the term "the optimum potency," meaning the potency on a plane most similar to that of the patient at the moment in question. Hahnemann's original choice of the word minimum served two purposes, first, to discourage the enormous crude drugging of his time, and secondly, to

12

point out that the high potencies have a different action from crude drugs. The whole potency question will be discussed in a later lecture in full.

The question of repeating the dose is the next in importance. As a simple rule for beginners high potencies should be given in one dose with *Placebo*; the low potencies, 30th and under, may need repetition. After giving the single dose of the single similar remedy the student *must watch and wait*. The duration of action of remedies and the factors influencing it will be discussed later. The general rule is to give nothing more than *Placebo* while improvement continues, in other words as long as the patient himself feels increasingly better regardless of the accentuation of certain symptoms. The beginner must learn not to try to make a good thing better by repetition as this defeats itself. According to the case, the potency, and the remedy, the need for repetition may occur in from a few hours in acute disease (to a few minutes in desperate cases) to weeks, months, and even a year or more in chronic cases, although waiting is perhaps the most difficult lesson for the eager homoeopath. He must wait with knowledge or valuable time will be wasted. How is he to know whether the remedy is the right one or is still acting? In acute cases the general well-being of the patient should be apparent in from a few moments to two or three days. In chronic cases it varies from a few hours to several weeks sometimes, indeed, it is only apparent after the second dose. In chronic cases Hering's law of cure, mentioned earlier in this paper, will show you whether you are on the right track. It is at this point, while watching the action of your remedy, that you must understand the subject of homoeopathic aggravations. An aggravation is not necessary to improvement, but it often occurs even with master prescribers. The usual cause of severe aggravation is an error in the potency or the presence of marked pathology. Aggravations are of two kinds, disease aggravation and remedy aggravation. The first of these is merely the natural progress of the disease and does not concern us here. The second or remedy aggravation, which is a sort of house-cleaning, is indicative of the prognosis of the case, and has about twelve recognizable forms which will be discussed later. Due allowance for aggravation must be made before considering repetition of the dose. A general rule is that even during aggravation, the patient, as a whole, in himself, feels better.

The subject of the second and subsequent prescriptions, one of the most important in the subject of homoeopathic philosophy, will be better understood in connection with prescribing later on.

Another very vital point in the homoeopathic philosophy is that of suppressions. The causation of suppressions is dependent on so many factors; the results of suppression untreated so dire, and frequently unrecognized; and the results treated so brilliant, that a complete lecture will be devoted to this subject.

To present homoeopathic philosophy lucidly and logically to a novice is well-nigh impossible. The student is urged to read and re-read the appended list of books.

READING LIST

Lectures on Homoeopathic Philosophy by James Tyler Kent, M.D.

The Genius of Homoeopathy by Stuart Close, M.D.

A Synopsis of Homoeopathic Philosophy by R. Gibson Miller, M.D., *Journal of Homoeopathists,* Vol. IV., August, 1900, page 194.

The Organon by Samuel Hahnemann, M.D.

Homoeopathy, the Science of Therapeutics by Carroll Dunham, M.D.

Manual of Pharmacodynamics by Richard Hughes, M.D.

KNOW THE PATIENT

"A case well taken is half cured," one of the masters said. For a good homoeopathic prescription a great deal of information is essential which is not needed in ordinary medicine. The homoeopath must know his patient, spiritually, emotionally, mentally, physically, and sociologically. He must give as much time as he needs to acquiring this knowledge. He must not prescribe anything but *Placebo*, in a chronic case, until he has it. In an acute case he must know these same factors in so far as they affect the acute condition. Let us suppose that a new patient comes into the office of a homoeopath. What is the procedure?

I. The physician must be receptive, like a photographic plate ready to receive the image of the patient. He must clear his mind of other preoccupations and of previous opinions about the patient. He must be tranquil, cordial, and after the first greeting and question, "What brings you to see me?" or "Tell me what it is that troubles you," he must be silent.

II. The physician must allow the patient to tell his own story in his own way. Questions or interruptions of any sort derail the patient at this stage, and may cause the doctor to lose essential information.

III. The physician must observe from the moment the patient enters. The office should be so arranged that the light falls on the patient. The main points to be noted are: (1) The personality of the patient. (2) His apparent state of mind both in himself and in relation to the doctor (whether depressed, shy, suspicious, secretive, afraid, ashamed, etc.). (3) His apparent physical status (signs of disease in gait, complexion, difficulty in breathing, etc.). (4) Traits of character as shown in dress, cleanliness, neatness, pride, etc.

IV. The physician must record every item which seems to him important, in the words of the patient, both in what the patient says and in what he himself observes, in a column at the left of his paper, leaving at least an inch blank between the items to be subsequently filled in as the patient reverts to that subject or later, when the physician questions about it. He may prefer to put facts pertaining to history on one sheet or in one column, those pertaining to actual physical symptoms in another, and mentals in a third, but this requires experience and adeptness. It is safer for the beginner to list them all as they come and sort them later in the working out of the case.

V. When the patient has come to a full stop the physician may say, "What else?" and by waiting elicit much more and often much more valuable information. If the patient is reticent or gives only brief and objective data, and the physician is unable to persuade him to give more, this passive method may have to be abandoned in favour of active questioning. The object is to drain the patient dry of what he knows of himself. If the patient is loquacious, time may necessitate the prevention of irrelevancies and the utmost tact is needed to keep him on the main track and yet not lose important sidelights.

VI. When the patient is through with his story a few remarks by the physician may be in order as to the aid that can be given though our remedies and the necessity for special knowledge of the patient as a whole and many details ordinarily overlooked. This pleases the patient and insures cooperation in answering the often rather intimate questions which must follow.

VII. The data needed for an ordinary medical history may hardly have been touched on up to this point and should not be inquired into even yet. If by this time the consultation period is over, if the patient is not in acute pain or distress, or has not come from a long distance, a subsequent appointment should be made for the next day if possible, and the patient should be definitely told that the physician must do a complete physical examination and the necessary routine laboratory tests at the next visit. Instructions for bringing a 24-hour urine specimen should then be given. This makes the patient realize that in addition to the interest to all details of the case the physician is going to be thoroughly scientific.

VIII. The physician should now take up each item that he has noted on paper and get the patient to tell him more about it. When the patient has exhausted all that he can tell about each item the physician should bring out the ''modalities;'' if, for instance, the item is pain in the stomach and the patient volunteers that it is burning and has no relation to meals and no radiation, the physician must find what aggravates or ameliorates it, what time it occurs, its concomitants, its relation to mental states, if any, etc. When each item has been so modified and filled in, the physician must run through the list and see which of the possible mentals, generals, particulars, and modalities have not been mentioned and question the patient about each of these.

IX. All questions that the physician asks must be so put that the patient cannot reply with a simple ''Yes'' or ''No'' but must think before answering. The physician must be careful never to suggest an answer by the form of his question and must guard against questioning for the symptoms of a particular remedy which may

17

have come to his mind. If he has seen a fairly definite remedy picture in the patient's story and wished to clinch it he must take special care not to lead the patient into the answer he desires, and may even suggest the opposite, and watch the reaction.

X. When the physician has covered the fields outlined above in detail, according to a systematic outline, which the novice should have before him during the interview and which the master knows by heart (we append a suggested one), he must make sure that he has questioned the patient on every system and function, otherwise some important detail will be missed which might prove a keynote suggesting the study of one or more remedies.

XI. The mental symptoms and characteristics of the patient (which, as will be brought out in a later lecture, are the most important if strongly marked) should usually be elicited last, when the patient's confidence has been more fully gained. Especial tact and insight on the part of the physician are needed to evaluate the emotional causes of disease; for instance, few patients would know that ailments from mortification might be the most important symptom in their cases, or that suppression of sex needs or anger might rank as a leading cause in their illness.

XII. At the close of the interview the patient must be made to feel that the physician is deeply interested in his case, that he will take the hours needed to thoroughly study up (to repertorize) the case, and that the special method of Homoeopathy can bring not only relief but also a fundamental improvement in the whole constitution which will tend to ward of subsequent illness and increase the powers and well-being of the patient. A thorough physical examination and the routine laboratory work, or any extra tests suggested by the history, must be done on every new patient and at least yearly on old patients, and the patients instructed as to why they should not use other drugs during homoeopathic treatment, what the dangers of suppression are, when they should report back, and what they may expect as the immediate results of the treatment. One other point may be valuable in knowing the patient and that is to get the version of the immediate family or close friends. This is sometimes dangerous, as nervous patients hate to know that they are being talked over, but the wise physician can take much contradictory evidence and arrive at a more just and sympathetic evaluation of the case.

By this time the physician should have a remarkably accurate picture of the patient in all his phases, subjective, objective, pathological. From this totality of symptoms he can, by correctly evaluating the symptoms as we will show in a subsequent lecture, derive a true image of the patient and the remedy.

OUTLINE FOR TAKING THE CASE

I. The patient's story
II. Modalities as applied to each of the above symptoms in the following order
   a. Causes
   b. Prodrome, onset, pace, sequence, duration
   c. Character, location, laterality, extension and radiation of pain or sensations
   d. Concomitants and alternations
   e. Aggravation or amelioration
      1. Time (hour, day, night, before or after midnight); periodicity; season; moon phases
      2. Temperature and weather: Chilly or warm-blooded usually, chilly or warm-blooded in present illness; wet, dry, cold, or hot weather; weather changes; storm or thunderstorm (before, during or after); hot sun, wind, fog, snow, open air, warm room, changes from one to other, stuffy or crowded places, drafts, warmth of bed, heat of stove, uncovering
      3. Bathing (hot, cold or sea), local applications (hot, cold, wet or dry)

19

4. Rest or motion (slow or rapid, ascending or descending, turning in bed, exertion, walking, on first motion, after moving a while, while moving, after moving), car and seasickness
5. Position: Standing, sitting, (knees crossed, rising from sitting), stooping (rising from stooping), lying (on painful side, back, right or left side, abdomen, head high or low, rising from lying), leaning head backward, forward, sidewise, closing or opening eyes, any unusual position such as knee-chest
6. External stimuli: Touch, hard or light, pressure, rubbing, constriction (clothing, etc.), jar, riding, stepping, light, noise, music, conversation, odors
7. Eating: In general (before, during, after, hot or cold food or drink), swallowing (solids, liquids, empty), acids, fats, salt, salty food, starches, sugar and sweets, green vegetables, milk, eggs, meat, fish, oysters, onions, beer, liquor, wine, coffee, tea, tobacco, drugs, etc.
8. Thirst, quantity, frequency, hot, cool or iced, sours, bitters, etc.
9. Sleep: In general (before, during, on falling asleep, in first sleep, after, on waking)
10. Menses (before, during, after, or suppressed)
11. Sweat: Hot or cold, foot-sweat, partial or suppressed
12. Other discharges: Bleeding, coryza, diarrhoea, vomitus, urine, emissions, leucorrhoea, etc.; suppression of same
13. Coition, continence, masturbation, etc.
14. Emotions: Anger, grief, mortification, fear, shock, consolation, apprehension of crowds, anticipation, suppression of same
f. Strange, rare and peculiar symptoms

III. The patient as a whole: *Mental Generals* (to be studied last for convenience), *Physical Generals*
PHYSICAL GENERALS
   a. The *constitutional type* of the patient (endo-crinologico-homoeopathic correspondences, lack or excess of vital heat, lack of reaction, sensitiveness, etc.)
   b. *Ailments from emotions* (see also mental generals); *suppressions* (emotions; discharges such as menses, sweat, leucorrhoea, catarrh, diarrhoea, etc.; eruptions; diseases such as malaria, rheumatic fever, exanthems, syphilis, gonorrhoea, etc.; of pathology such as haemorrhoids, fistulae, ulcers, tonsils, tumors, other surgical conditions, etc.); from *exposure* to cold, wet, hot sun, etc.; from *mechanical conditions* such as overeating, injury, etc.
   c. *Menses*, date of establishment, regularity (early or late), duration, color, consistency, odor, amount, clots, membrane, pain (modalities of), concomitants, aggravation or amelioration before, during, or after, both physically and mentally, menopause (symptoms of)
   d. Other *discharges* (see II. e. 12) cause, color, consistency, odor, acrid or bland, symptoms from suppression of, symptoms alternating with, hot or cold, partial discharges as of sweat, laterality, better or worse from discharges (before, during, or after)
   e. *Sleep*, better or worse from, position in, aggravation after, difficulty in getting to sleep, waking frequently or early, at what hour, somnambulism, talking in sleep, dreams (see Mentals), restless during
   f. *Restlessness, prostration, weakness, trembling, chill, fever*, etc.
   g. *Aggravations* and *ameliorations* applying to patient as a whole as under II. e. 1 to 14.

21

h. *Objective symptoms* such as redness of orifices, superfluous hair, applying to patient as a whole
i. *Pathology* which applies to patient as a whole, such as tendency to tumors, wens, cysts, polyps, warts, moles, individual and family tendency to certain diseases or weaknesses of specific organs or tissues (also related to a. above and to physical examination), frequency of catching cold

MENTAL GENERALS

a. *Will:* Loves, hates, and emotions (suicidal, loathing of life; lasciviousness, revulsion to sex, sexual perversions; fears; greed, eating, money, emotionality, smoking, drinking, drugs; dreams; homicidal tendencies, desire or aversion to company, family, friends; jealousy, suspicion, obstinacy, contrariness, depression, loquacity, weeping, laughing, impatience, conscientiousness)

b. *Understanding:* Delusions, delirium, hallucinations, mental confusion, loss of time sense

c. *Intellect:* Memory, concentration, mistakes in writing and speaking

IV. Quick review of condition of every system and organ, beginning with head and following order of Kent's *Repertory*

V. Past history of patient in seven-year periods

VI. Family history

VII. Physical examination and laboratory tests.

KNOW THE REMEDIES

Theoretically any substance or force may become a homoeopathic remedy. In a large number of instances of so-called physiologically inert substances in the crude state, varying degrees of potentization are necessary to bring out the remedial powers. At present no complete list of all homoeopathic remedies exists. At a rough guess some two or three thousand remedies are in use and new ones are continually being developed. Only a relatively small number of these are thoroughly proved according to the Hahnemannian standard, and but few according to a modern scientific homoeopathic standard. The remedies in accepted use are divided for convenience into certain groups as follows: (1) Mineral remedies, including elements, metals, compounds, salts, etc. (2) Vegetable remedies. (3) Animal remedies. (4) The nosodes, which are remedies derived from morbid tissues and secretions. (5) Sarcodes, which are remedies prepared from healthy animal tissues and secretions, such as *Uric Acid* and *Thyro-iodine*. This also includes endocrine remedies. (6) Imponderabilia, which include positive and negative magnetic force, electricity, sun force, etc.

The information about these remedies is obtained from the following sources: from provings, which means experimentation on the relatively healthy; from toxicology, which contributes the extreme symptoms and in part the pathology; from experimentation on animals, organs and tissues in the laboratory; from clinical verification of symptoms by cure; from clinical appearance of remedy symptoms during medication; and from human pathology which has been cured. The main classical source of the knowledge of remedies is, of course, the proving. The subject of how to make correct provings and standardize them is an important one, but it does not come in under this elementary course.

Now we come to actual methods of acquiring and retaining the general picture and detailed knowledge of this bevy of remedies. This is no simple task as anyone reading the proving of a polychrest, such as *Calcarea*, will realize. No mind can retain such a mass of symptoms which often seem unrelated and contradictory. *One must learn how to study a remedy.*

The most important thing to get in the study of a remedy is the feel of it. The essence of Homoeopathy being individualization, and each well-proved drug having a definite personality, the student must get acquainted with the different remedies in the materia medica as if they were friends. He must be able to recognize them from partial expressions even when he cannot see the whole picture, as he would know a well-known person in a group across the room. Experts in prescribing are so saturated with the remedies that they can often choose them intuitively and although this is dangerous to the beginner it should be the goal of all.

We suggest the following plan for systematic remedy study:

For those who do not contact humans in this way, and indeed for all at first, the study of a remedy must begin with a knowledge of its mentals. The innermost of man being the most important, the psychic characteristics and peculiarities of each remedy individual must be thoroughly mastered. You could not conceive of giving *Sulphur* as a chronic remedy to a woman in whose linen closet the towels and napery were tied neatly with rose-colored ribbon. You would not give

Phosphorus to one who was abnormally modest, nor *Arsenicum* to a sloven. Unfortunately many of our remedies have not a fully-developed proving of mental symptoms, but where these exist they are of prime importance.

Many more drugs have clearly-marked modalities, in other words aggravation from or amelioration by meteorological conditions and such things as motion, heat, jar, touch, position, classes of foods, or special substances, etc. The marked desires and aversions, aggravations and ameliorations, should become etched on the mind of the student, both those which affect the personality as a whole, and those, often agreeing but sometimes contradictory, which modify the affected part.

Of particular importance, in the knowledge of materia medica, and often difficult to find in books, are the causations of disease typical of the different remedies. These may be mental or general. The student should pay particular attention to the symptoms of ailments from emotion (such as mortification in *Staphisagria;* anger in *Chamomilla, Colocynth, Nux vomica;* grief in *Ignatia;* fright in *Aconite*, etc.) and also to ailments from injury *(Arnica, Natrum sulph.)*. Ailments from suppressed discharges are of paramount importance, whether they be from mucous membranes, such as leucorrhoea, diarrhoea, etc. or from the skin as in the case of perspiration or eruptions, or from operations which close nature's vents, such as fistulae or haemorrhoids. The fourth important variety of causation is that due to chilling of various kinds, non-mechanical dietary indiscretions, etc., these being applicable more frequently in acute diseases.

When the student has mastered the various points about the remedy he should study the localities of the body to which the remedy especially applies, and make a chart of a figure with the vulnerable points of the remedy suitably drawn in. In this connection he would do well to make a diagram of the tongue, its condition often being characteristic and giving valuable hints for prescribing. He may also make drawings of different parts of the body such as the eyes, representing the various conditions in those organs cured by the remedy. These schemata aid memory by visualization. Not only the organ influenced by a remedy should be learned, but also the tissues, as for instance that *Bryonia* is suitable to inflammation of serous membranes, where *Belladonna* is rarely so.

The student should then pick out from among the welter of particular symptoms those which are "strange, rare, and peculiar," the so-called "keynotes" of the remedy, and have these at his fingers' ends as signposts to point the way to further study. In this connection he should pick out similes from literature (such as the analogy between the precocious *Lycopodium* child and Paul Dombey) and expressive epithets (such as "mince-pie fiend"—*Carbo veg.*, the "human barometer"—*Rhus tox.*, "gloomy Gus"—*Natrum carb.*, the "false ragged philosopher"—*Sulphur*, etc.).

He should pay especial attention to the pictures of acute disease in chronic remedies and to the different types of chronic personality in each remedy.

He should get clearly in mind the important details relating to the bodily functions such as menstruation, pregnancy, digestion, sleep, and excretion, whether by skin, bowels, or urinary tract.

He should make a remedy clock, a diagram showing the time of general aggravation and special aggravations of the remedy in question.

Picking out the alternating conditions and the concomitant conditions, and keeping them clearly in mind is of great help, although rarely done. (The second edition of Kent's *Repertory* has a separate heading for alternations, which, in the third edition, are sprinkled through the book). It will be very helpful to the beginner to make a note of the main contradictions in symptoms in each remedy and to think through why this should be so.

By this time the student is in a position to note, without danger of being unduly influenced by pathology, the different "diseases" in which the remedy under study is especially useful; and after thoroughly mastering the polychrests he should go back and compare their action in each of the diseases. Very little has been written anywhere about comparisons between the physiological action of drugs and their homoeopathic action, but in the study of each remedy its pharmacology and uses in regular medicine should be looked up and compared. Useful hints and analogies are often forthcoming.

The student should correlate the homoeopathic remedy picture with endocrinology, metabolic tests and morphology.

Study one polychrest each week, beginning with relatively easy ones such as *Aconite, Belladonna, Bryonia,* and then, when the habit of assimilating the remedy is acquired, tackle the essential drugs, such as *Sulphur, Calcarea, Silica, Phosporus,* etc.

Each remedy should be studied in at least ten different books so as to allow for the refractions of the personalities of the different authors. No human being sees all aspects of another individual or of a drug. A composite picture is necessary to completeness. We would recommend the following books for study in the order mentioned:

Kent's *Materia Medica,* which, though informal in style, gives a compelling and permeating picture of the remedies.

Nash's *Leaders,* a dangerous book if used alone, but stimulating and comprehensive.

Allen's *Keynotes,* in a class with the above.

Clarke's *Dictionary of Materia Medica,* not the symptoms of the provings themselves, but the "characteristics" which give interesting varied information and sparse salient features.

Hering's *Guiding Symptoms,* with especial attention

to the symptoms with heavy and double heavy marks, this being the most solid and practicable of all our materia medicas, although it does not give the picturesque individuality of the drugs as Kent does.

Dunham's *Lectures on Materia Medica*, very lucid.

Hahnemann's *Materia Medica Pura*, the prime source of the subject, placed late on the list because of the mass of symptoms.

Teste's *Materia Medica*, giving suggestive groupings of the remedies, a unique book.

Allen's *Encyclopaedia of the Materia Medica*, difficult reading because of the mass of material, but invaluable.

Jahr's *Manual*, which has many symptoms not to be found elsewhere.

When the nosodes are studied, H. C. Allen's *Materia Medica of the Nosodes* should be added, and for unusual remedies Kent's *Lesser Writings*, Hale's *New Remedies*, and Anshutz's *New, Old, and Forgotten Remedies*. For those who read German, Stauffer's *Homöopathische Arzneimittellehre*, as yet untranslated, is a classic.

The student should also read Farrington's *Clinical Materia Medica* although it is confusing, and Hughes' *Manual*, or better his *Cyclopaedia of Drug Pathogenesy*, Cowperthwaite's *Materia Medica*, Pierce's *Plain Talks on Materia Medica for Nurses*, Rabe's *Therapeutics*, and Boger's *Synoptic Key*.

The student would do well before finishing his study to outline the emergency uses of each of the remedies and commit them to memory.

As a check to his study he can take the Kent *Repertory* and run through for the rubrics in which the remedy he is studying appears in the third (highest) degree.

If the student will follow this outline and get the habit of recognizing remedy types in street cars, at meetings, wherever he may be, his knowledge will be solid and broad, and his time saved.

THE EVALUATION OF SYMPTOMS

In the lecture on case taking we gave, in some detail, the hierarchy of the symptoms, and would suggest that, in connection with this article, the reader reperuse that one. The evaluation of symptoms is, perhaps, the most important part of the homoeopathic technique, and to the beginner, one of the most difficult. Certain propositions in relation to it are axiomatic. Owing to the terminology of modern medicine and the training that patients have received from non-homoeopathic physicians, the emphasis which the patient himself places upon symptoms is often entirely misleading. The doctor must separate diagnoses and common symptoms (that is symptoms which are common to any patient suffering from a certain complaint, such as vomiting in a gastro-intestinal case). *These common symptoms* are valueless from the point of view of homoeopathic prescribing unless qualified by modalities. The physician must discriminate between the relatively worthless common symptoms, which may often be the patient's chief complaint, and the precious minor, subjective symptoms which the patient, inadvertently, brings out. The patient may complain loud and long of some pain or inconvenience which is relatively irrelevant, and not even be aware of grave and helpful symptoms plain to the physician.

On the other hand, just because the physician knows that mental symptoms are most important he should not hunt in the haystack for a tiny mental, with which to open his case. *The symptoms should have the same*

29

importance, the same weight or mass, in the patient's case as is assigned to them in the symptom hierarchy. For example, a woman complains of indigestion and admits to overpowering fears; the fears, being a mental, outrank the symptoms: but if this woman had violent pain in the stomach and an unimportant fear, the pain being a much greater factor in the case, would outrank the fear.

A third axiom is that all rubrics used, or rather symptoms taken to be matched with rubrics, must be really true of the patient and reliable.

Another is that three or more similar particulars make a general, for instance, if the patient has burning in the head, the stomach, the feet and the skin the general rubric *burning* is applicable; whereas, if he has burning in the stomach only, it is a particular.

If a valuable general cannot be found in the *Repertory*, as stated by the patient, it may be found under the opposite rubric, as, "cold weather ameliorates." This is found in the *Repertory* under "warm air aggravates." "Better in summer" is found under "winter aggravates." This again brings up the nice problem of the interpretation of the terms of the rubrics. Only a knowledge of the exact meaning of words and of psychology sufficient to divine what the patient means by what he says, and a thorough acquaintance with every rubric in the *Repertory*, will enable the physician to allocate symptoms.

If care and ingenuity are taken it is not only justifiable, but sometimes necessary, to combine rubrics in order to get the exact meaning. There are two ways of combining, by adding all the remedies in the two or more rubrics, especially when the rubrics are small; or taking only the remedies which appear in all the rubrics taken, which increases the grading of the remedies. An example of rubrics which may be combined by this latter method is, menses, acrid, early, bright red, and clotted.

There is divergence of opinion as to the proper place

of pathology and also of objective symptoms (such as redness of the orifices). In the Kentian method, these are placed relatively low, whereas the Boger method, as given in his little *General Analysis,* stresses the pathological generals, as opposed to diagnostic pathology. Stearns favors stressing the objective symptoms as he feels that these cannot mislead.

There are several kinds of pathology. Disease diagnoses appear here and there in the *Repertory,* as, scarlet fever, septicemia, chorea, apoplexy, etc. Other conditions which are pathological and yet are symptoms rather than diseases are found, such as convulsions dropsy, cyanosis, haemorrhage, etc. There is a third class of pathology, the importance of which consists in the bodily tendency to produce such changes, such as, warts, polypi, fibroid tumours, etc. These are the most important of the pathological rubrics as they indicate the tendency of the whole constitution. Such a rubric as empyema, which is found under chest, is a pathological particular and less important although it may be of great interest in such a case to see what remedies have had the power to cause and to cure this condition.

The schema of the order of importance of symptoms according to Kent is:

Mentals—will, understanding, intellect.

Physical generals—time, temperature, weather, position, motion, external stimuli, eating, drinking, sleep, clothing, and bathing.

Particulars—strange, rare, and peculiar, and the modalities of the particulars.

In the Kent method after taking the complete case the physician selects any outstanding mentals, grading them in the order above given. He, of course, adds such mentals as he, himself, perceives in the patient or as a cause of the ailment. There may be from one, or indeed none, to six or seven marked mentals. The physician then takes the chief generals in the case, ranking them in the order above given. The mentals plus the generals will give him a working basis for the selection of a chronic remedy. When the physician has repertorized these symptoms down to about five remedies he should then rank the particulars and see how the five remedies cover these. Then he must take these five remedies and study them in the materia medica, in order to select the one most similar to the case. It is obvious that this method proceeds from generals to particulars, and no special attention is paid to pathology.

In the Boger method fewer symptoms are used and special stress is put on pathological generals, for instance if the case presents several excoriating discharges the rubric Acridity, in Boger's *General Analysis,* would be taken; if the patient complains of marked dryness of mouth, rectum, skin, etc., the general *Dryness* would be used. In this method the mentals are prominent and take first place, as in the Kent method.

Stearns takes not more than five or six symptoms, of which one is mental, one pathological, one objective and two physical generals.

Boericke divides symptoms into basic and determinative classes, the basic being the common, diagnostic and pathologic; and the determinative the subjective, modalities, and generals. Boericke, like Dr. Margaret Tyler, in England, advocates the use of certain large general rubrics, such as lack of vital heat, as eliminative symptoms, which some Kentians consider dangerous.

It is hoped that the student will not be confused by this variance of method among the masters and it is strongly recommended that each beginner master the Kentian technique first, the other variants being shortcuts to suit different types of minds.

As soon as the case is taken and the physician sits down to study it, he will find it useful to run down the list of symptoms and mark with M opposite the mentals, G opposite the generals, PATH opposite the pathology, P opposite the particular and O for objectives.

This should be done in the left hand margin and should be in a colored pencil. For further clarity he may underline any peculiar symptoms in red. The symptoms to be actually used for repertorizing should be written off on a new sheet in the order of their importance. If the Kent method is being used he is then ready to transcribe the symptoms into the special blank repertory sheets which can be purchased from the American Foundation of Homoeopathy and which greatly simplify repertorizing.

After the beginner has listed his symptoms according to their importance he should reconsider, checking mentally his symptom list with his impression of the patient and see if any elements of the case are placed too high or too low; for on the correct evaluation of the symptoms depends the possibility of finding the most similar remedy which will lead to cure.

REPERTORIZING

As no one person can carry all the symptoms of all the remedies in his mind, a concordance or index is needed. We term a symptom index a repertory. There are about half a hundred of these, general or special, based on different systems of studying the case. The two most vital to know are the basic ones of the two main methods, the Kent *Repertory* and the Boenninghausen.

THE KENT REPERTORY: ITS CONSTRUCTION

The Kent *Repertory* is a compilation of materia medica, certain prior repertories, such as Lippe's, and clinical symptoms verified. In order to successfully search in the Kent *Repertory* for the symptoms of your case as evaluated in accordance with our last lecture you must be thoroughly familiar with the plan of the book, its rationale, and also its inconsistencies. The plan of the book is to work from generals to particulars, a general rubric first in most instances. The book is based on anatomical divisions, (see Table of Contents, p. VII), with certain exceptions such as the first section on MIND; the last one, GENERALITIES; discharges, such as STOOL, SWEAT, URINE, and EXPEC-TORATION, which appear as separate sections next to the anatomical region producing them; and certain general conditions, such as VERTIGO, COUGH, SLEEP, CHILL, and FEVER, which are also separate. Under each anatomical section the rubrics run in alphabetical order regardless of whether they are pathology, sensations, modalities, or objective symptoms (such as "bores head in pillow", page 108). Each such main heading is followed by modifiers (if there be such), in the order following: time, circumstances in alphabetical order, extensions (the point *from* which a symptom extends is the one under which it will be found, not the point *to* which it extends), location with *its* time, circumstance and extension modifiers, and lastly, sensation with its modifiers. For instance, the main section HEAD is anatomical, but under that you will *not* find an anatomical section for occiput, rather must you look under the sensation in the occiput, as for instance, *Coldness or Pain, Occiput, in*.

It is to be noted that certain anatomical regions have no corresponding section in this *Repertory*, for instance, NECK, which is found under THROAT, EXTERNAL THROAT, and BACK. EXTERNAL THROAT contains the rubrics pertaining to the anterior neck, such as goitre, glands, torticollis, etc., and BACK contains nape and posterior cervical region. Furthermore lungs, heart, aorta, axillary glands, breast, and milk appear under CHEST; posterior chest appears under BACK; pulse under GENERALITIES; head sinuses are divided between NOSE and FACE; salivary glands are found under FACE instead of under THROAT; lips under FACE instead of under THROAT, MOUTH; oesophagus is found under STOMACH; and liver under ABDOMEN. There is no section for the circulatory, glandular, or nervous systems, as this book is not based on systems (Boericke's *Repertory* is in part), but the parts of these systems are found scattered throughout the book under allied anatomical headings. Many symptoms which one would expect to find under the nervous system appear under GENERALITIES as they indicate a tendency of the whole organism, such as Analgesia, Chorea, Convulsions, Paralysis, Trembling, etc. Twitching of the parts appears under the anatomical part, such as FACE, EXTREMITIES. Nervous symptoms having to do with the spine appear under BACK, such as *Opisthotonos*. Meningitis appears in two places, under HEAD, *Inflammation*, meninges of, and BACK, *Inflammation*, cord, membranes of.

Similar or allied rubrics often appear in two or more different places, as for instance; Dysmenorrhoea under GENITALIA, FEMALE, *Menses* painful; ABDOMEN, *Pain*, cramping, bearing down, cutting, menses, during; ABDOMEN, *Pain*, hypogastrium, in, menses, during; and ABDOMEN, *Pain*, menses, during.

It must be noted that many rubrics which appear as particulars under the proper anatomical sections or main headings also appear in the last section, GENERALITIES, in their relation to the body as a whole; for instance, under GENERALITIES, *Menses,* comes aggravation or amelioration of the whole person before, during or after menses, while under GENITALIA FEMALE appears the type and circumstances of the menses, or, so to speak, the particulars. Similarly under GENERALITIES, *Perspiration,* appears amelioration or aggravation of the body as a whole from sweat, whereas under the section PERSPIRATION are given the quality, occurrence, and modalities of the discharge itself. Sweat of any especial part is found under the anatomical section in which the part is located, such as, ABDOMEN, *Perspiration* on. Perspiration of the scalp is not under HEAD, scalp, perspiration of, but under HEAD, *Perspiration*, scalp of. General amelioration by, or distress from, the act of eating appears under GENERALITIES, *Eating;* and under GENERALITIES, *Food,* are the aggravations and ameliorations from the different articles of food, but under the section STOMACH, aversions and desires for special articles of food appear.

Pathological diagnoses are found frequently in GENERALITIES and occasionally as headings under other sections but more often as subheadings, under the condition involved; for instance, pleurisy is found under CHEST, *Inflammation*, pleura of, and appendicitis under ABDOMEN, *Inflammation*, appendicitis. On the other hand empyema is found under CHEST, *Empyema*, directly, and goitre under EXTERNAL THROAT, *Goitre*. Certain pathological states which are symptoms rather than diseases, such as *Chorea, Convulsions, Cyanosis, Dropsy*, etc., appear under GENERALITIES. Objective symptoms are scattered all through the book and are often small unclassified rubrics, such as *Brittle Nails, Gestures* under MIND, *Biting* under MIND, and red lips under FACE, *Discoloration*, red lips.

THE KENT REPERTORY: ITS USE

This *Repertory* is built to work the cases from general symptoms to particular symptoms. We have already spoken in our lecture on the evaluation of symptoms of Kent's method of grading, MENTALS being the most important, and GENERALS next. Most chronic cases and many acute ones can be worked out by the *Repertory* on the MENTALS and GENERALS alone to within three to five remedies. The beginner should take at least eight of these symptoms, although experts often solve the case on three to five. The beginner must be very sure that these MENTALS and GENERALS are really true of the patient, and that he has not warped the symptom in translating the patient's colloquial expressions into the language of the rubrics. Moreover a symptom must have the same mass or importance in the patient's case as is assigned to it in the symptom hierarchy. If an important symptom cannot be found in the *Repertory* it can often be found under a synonymous rubric. It is to be understood that the headings under GENERALITIES which are not pathological and not marked "ameliorated by," or otherwise explained, and which are not sensations or conditions mean "aggravation from," for example, *Eating*, before, means worse before eating, *Coition*, after, means aggravated after coition, etc. Many of the ameliorations are omitted and you must look for them under aggravation under their opposites; for instance, there is no better in summer. This is considered equivalent to worse in winter. Sometimes two or more rubrics must be combined in order to be equivalent to a given symptom. If the rubrics are very small it may be wise to add all the remedies. If at least one of the rubrics is large and the others fair size, only such remedies as run through all the component rubrics of this symptom should be taken. Certain symptoms have so large a group of remedies that they are almost useless except as eliminating symptoms. Such a one is cold-bloodedness of the patient, which appears under GENERALITIES, *Heat*, lack of vital, and would serve to eliminate any markedly hot-blooded remedies which had otherwise come through the generals high in a given case.

The student will recall from our previous lecture that the common symptoms, or the unqualified big, main rubrics, such as Sadness, Vomiting, etc., are of little or no use in repertorizing, and that among both GENERALS and PARTICULARS, a strange, rare, and peculiar symptom ranks high. A strange, rare, and peculiar general would be "during cold stage craves cold", or "during hot stage craves heat", as in *Camphor;* a strange, rare, and peculiar particular would be "thirst for ice water only during chill" *(Eup. per.).*

We have said that the beginner should locate in the *Repertory* his eight or more main GENERALS and chart the remedies appearing under each of these, putting 3 for the bold face (heavy black type), 2 for italics, and 1 for roman (plain type); this being done for all the

38

symptoms chosen, the remedies appearing in more than half the rubrics are listed with their fractions, the numerator of the fraction being the numerical totality of the remedy grades, and the denominator being the number of symptoms in which the remedy appears. Now the PARTICULARS come into play, beginning with the most peculiar ones, and care should be taken not to use too small rubrics. In fact it is safer to use a more general, medium-sized rubric than the more exact particular rubric. The occurrence of these particulars in the few remedies which have stood highest in the GENERALS, and in these only, being taken, you can now see which few remedies are fairly similar to the GENERALS of your case, and which few of those most resemble the PARTICULARS of the case. Add the particular to the general fraction and reduce your list to the three or five remedies which stand highest in their grand total. If one remedy totals 16/7 and another 15/8, the former is to be preferred. As you have taken your symptoms in the strict order of their importance according to the Kentian schema your first two or three symptoms should appear in the remedies that come high, and where they do not the remedy should be looked on with suspicion. It is to be remembered that certain remedies, like *Sulph.*, *Calc.*, *Nux*, *Puls.*, etc. almost always come out high numerically because they have been so thoroughly proved, and unless the beginner discounts this and bases his final judgment on materia medica and especially the mentals and type of the patient he will prescribe these well-proved polychrests too often. Conversely, it must not be forgotten that some remedies, like *Tub.*, have but a fragmentary part of their proving in the *Repertory*, and that only a little more than 500 remedies are mentioned in the *Repertory*, and very few of the nosodes and double salts are adequately stressed. When the remedies have been reduced numerically to from three to five, these must be read in the materia medicas, especially their MENTALS, and the original case as taken reviewed and compared to each of the remedies. The miasmatic relationships of the patient and of the remedies that come out high must be considered. For future reference in treating the case, in acute as well as chronic prescribing, a list should be made on the chart of the constitutional remedies which come high, of the nosodes which most nearly apply, and of the acute remedies ranking highest. These, or complements of these, will often be found to fit any illness of that patient in the future, unless an epidemic remedy be called for.

Ideally, on the repertorizing record each symptom should be stated in the words of the patient in the symptom column, restated in the exactly corresponding rubric in the rubric column, and the page where this is found after it. There are repertorizing sheets on graph paper with the main remedies printed in, numbered places for writing in symptoms, etc., which are a great convenience and a time saver.

THE BOENNINGHAUSEN REPERTORY:
ITS CONSTRUCTION

Boenninghausen's *Therapeutic Pocket Book*, one of the earliest repertories, is based largely on Hahnemann's *Materia Medica Pura* and the idea of it was approved by Hahnemann himself. The book falls into seven distinct parts. Although each of these is complete in itself, "yet each one gives but one portion of a symptom, which can be completed only in one or several other parts." For example, the seat of pain is found in the second section, the kind of pain in the third, the aggravation or amelioration according to time or circumstances in the sixth, and the necessary concomitants in the various sections. The seven sections are: 1. The Mind and Disposition; 2. Parts of the Body and Organs; 3. Sensations and Complaints in alphabetical order, in general and then specially, of the glands, of the bones, and of the skin and exterior parts; 4. Sleep and Dreams; 5. Fevers with Chill, Circulation and Sweat (the 2nd, 4th, and 5th sections have concomitants); 6. Aggravations and Ameliorations from time and circumstances; 7. Relationship of Remedies. In section seven under each drug the previous section headings, 1 through 6, are given and under each the remedies applying in that section which are related to the drug in question. At the end of each drug is given a list of other related remedies and the antidotes.

THE BOENNINGHAUSEN REPERTORY: ITS USE

This Repertory is based on GENERALS even much more than the Kent. The rubrics in the different sections dealing with the different aspects of one symptom are used to eliminate all remedies but such as run through them all. This is a swifter, easier method than the Kent, but too general, and a great many symptoms cannot be found in it at all. Also there are very few rubrics under MIND, only seven pages out of 482. Boger's *General Analysis* is based on this repertory and his unique method of working cases by it is also deserving of study.

THE BOERICKE REPERTORY

The Kent *Repertory* in its present form is unwieldy for the physician to carry with him to the bedside. Neither the Boenninghausen nor Kent repertories have any materia medica. Two books which combine materia medica and repertory are handy in the pocket or medical bag. One of these is Boger's *Synoptic Key,* of which his *General Analysis* is an abridged form, and the other is Boericke's *Materia Medica with Repertory.* The Boericke *Repertory* resembles the Kent rather than the Boenninghausen but Boericke has reclassified some of the anatomical sections. For instance, vertigo appears under HEAD; sinuses are grouped together under NOSE; lips are under MOUTH instead of FACE; TONGUE has a section to

41

itself as have GUMS; oesophagus is under THROAT instead of STOMACH; foods that disagree are in STOMACH with the cravings and aversions; rectum and stool are under ABDOMEN; all the URINARY SYSTEM is together under that heading; breasts are rightly classed under the FEMALE SEXUAL SYSTEM; there is an admirable section on Pregnancy, Labor and Lactation; after genitalia comes the section on the CIRCULATORY SYSTEM including pulse; then comes the LOCOMOTOR SYSTEM including extremities, gait, neck, inflammatory rheumatism and arthritis, back, and axillae; then comes RESPIRATORY SYSTEM, including lungs, cough, expectoration, larynx, voice, and respiration; following this is the SKIN. The FEVER section includes chill and sweat, the exanthems, and various fevers such as influenza, typhoid, malaria, etc. The NERVOUS SYSTEM follows and includes epilepsy, paralysis, sleep, dreams, weakness, convulsions, goitre, sea-sickness, neuralgia, sciatica, spine, meningitis, etc. The GENERALITIES section is much reduced and contains mainly diseases, tissues, poisonings, suppressions (under Checked discharges), glandular affections including mumps, goitre, a very interesting section on Complaints: from winds, damp places, sudden, gradual, injuries, prophylactics, and tumors. This section has been relieved of much misplaced matter and has added to it a great deal of interesting and valuable material. The last section is MODALITIES, first aggravations and then ameliorations, and time under these appears in alphabetical order under morning, night, periodicity, etc., instead of all together at the beginning of the section as in Kent.

Under all extensive headings, such as Headache, appear definite captions in the following order: Cause, Type, Location, Character of Pain, Concomitants, Modalities, i. e. Aggravations and Ameliorations.

This book is a clinical rather than a symptomatological index and has many technical terms as main headings. A tremendous number of remedies are given in the materia medica section, and well given, with plentiful mentals. Owing to its small size a great many symptoms have had to be omitted from the repertory. Its pretensions are not great but its usefulness within its sphere is tremendous.

This gives the beginner a bird's eye view of three of the most useable general repertories. It is strongly advised that every student master the Kent method, as it will reward familiarity more than any other. To the advanced student it should be added that many strange and peculiar symptoms cannot be found in these three repertories and must be searched for in Gentry's *Concordance,* Knerr's *Repertory,* Lippe, Jahr, or some of the special repertories.

Card repertories have not been mentioned. There is one by Field, based largely on the Kent, but inaccurate. It is useful for hurried, acute prescribing in the office. A new card repertory, exactly following Kent, is now under construction by the Doctors Pulford of Toledo, Ohio. Boger's cards closely follow his *Synoptic Key.*

These different methods of repertorizing will appeal to different types of minds and will also be suitable for different types of cases: the Boger method suiting those with much pathology and few other symptoms; the Kent method suiting those with marked mentals and an intricate anamnesis; the Boenninghausen suiting conditions with acute pains and clear-cut modalities, cases without subtleties. In closing this brief, suggestive method of repertory study we would reiterate, STUDY THE KENT METHOD FIRST, LAST, AND ALL THE TIME.

PRESCRIBING:

POTENCY SELECTION

After thoroughly digesting the first six lectures of this brief course and doing wide collateral reading and studying one should be able to select the most similar remedy. The most similar remedy, however, does not become the *similimum* until the potency is adjusted to the plane of the individual during his or her illness at the time of prescribing. Our philosophy teaches us that pathology, and even bacteria, are ultimates of disease and that the true cause is far deeper and less material than these. In order to truly wipe out the cause of a so-called disease one must administer the remedy on or near the plane of the cause. It follows that for mental distresses and disease of manifestly psychic origin the high potencies (10 M and upward) would be employed, other things being equal; and that for grossly material conditions, such as marked organic and pathologic changes, the lower or medium potencies would be selected. In general, then, functional diseases, where the symptoms are subjective or physiological, where the vital force is tactile, respond well to high potencies; and the organic conditions to lower ones. It makes some difference whether the conditon be acute or chronic. For instance, diphtheria has marked pathology, as has pneumonia, yet the pathology in diphtheria is recent and swift in pace, and the high potencies are suitable. In general, acute diseases respond well to high potencies, especially of acute remedies (high potencies of deep-acting chronic remedies, when these are indicated in an acute condition, may be dangerous). Certain acute crises, based on chronic trouble, such as cardiac asthma, would have to be treated with medium or low potencies because the high potency would stir up more than the vital force could cope with in the face of the advanced chronic pathology.

In chronic prescribing it is a safe rule to begin with the 200th centesimal unless this is dangerous because of the nature of the remedy, the degree of the pathology, or the depth of the miasms. One great object in starting at the 200th in chronic cases is that you then have an ascending series of potencies to use as treatment progresses. The Kentian ideal is to exhaust the action of one potency (see section on *Repetition* below) and then to step up to the next, exhaust that, and so on, if no change of remedy is indicated, to the highest potency known of that remedy. (Hahnemann places the upper limit of potencies suitable at the end of a series in any given case at the last potency which will produce a very slight aggravation of the symptoms. In our experience you can usually use the highest known potency of the *similimum* and still get action, although at times action will cease with, say the CM potency). When the top of the series has been exhausted and the same remedy is still called for you begin again at the 200th and repeat the ascending series.

Series of homoeopathic potencies have been made by many famous persons, either by hand, as in the case of the Jenichen potencies, or by various machines. As a general rule it is best to stick to the potencies made by one man as you go up the series in any one case, as for instance, Kent's 200th, 1M, 10M, CM, etc.. On the other hand, if a jolt is needed, although the same remedy is called for, a change from, say the Skinner to the Fincke potencies may whip up the case. For those who understand rhythms and cycles it may be well, after a patient has been through a course (ascending series) of a remedy from one source, to change to one of the irregular potencies of the remedy from another source; for instance, we have seen Skinner's *Lyc*. 2M beneficial instead of Kent's 1M, or Fincke's 43M in place of a 50M. This change seems to start a new rhythm or cycle, it is as though the vital force became bored with the decimal system and responded with a renewed spurt to the alteration of potency. This is advanced doctrine.

In desperately ill cases, where the fight for life is active, in acute disease, the high potencies are indicated; also, where the desperate illness is the terminal stage of chronic disease, the very high potencies induce euthanasia. In chronically incurable cases, unless the vitality is very good and the pathology not yet too extreme, low or medium potencies are suitable, and usually the deep-acting *similimum* must here be avoided and a palliative drug given. If such a palliative be not too searching a remedy, *(Sang., Rumex, Puls.,)* etc., it may be given even to incurables in a fairly high potency.

The problem of potency selection in acute disease incident to chronic treatment is another snag. Patients long under correct chronic prescribing show fewer and fewer acute diseases. In other words their susceptibility is eradicated. However, explosions of latent psora do occur sometimes, particularly when the vigor is increased by the proper chronic remedy, as a sort of vent or effort on the part of the vital force towards house-cleaning. The first problem for the prescriber in this connection is to determine whether the acute symptoms arising during chronic treatment are an aggravation following the remedy, and if so, whether they are an aggravation due to the reactive curative power of the body, or a remedy aggravation due to over-sensitivity, or to *wrong potency*. If either of these be the case and the aggravation is not too severe no remedy should be given, merely *Placebo*. If the aggravation threatens life or is unbearably painful (this may have to be antidoted) or, for some social reason, particularly intolerable for the moment, an acute remedy may be given in the medium-low potencies, preferably the 30th or 200th, and this will probably not interfere with the action of the chronic remedy. In acute exacerbations or explosions of active chronic disease you can often give the acute complement or cognate of your chronic remedy. In this case also the chronic remedy may continue to act undisturbed. In very severe acute diseases during the course of chronic treatment it will sometimes be better to give the acute remedy high, and, after the acute condition has subsided, *retake* the chronic case, which will often show a new picture. The new prescription takes into account the original chronic symptoms but lays more stress on the recent developments.

In many conditions with marked tissue change, such as adhesions, chronic cardiac decompensation, very low potencies, even tinctures, may be useful. Potencies as low as the 12th or even the 6th are occasionally invaluable in single doses in such grave conditions as tuberculosis, where even a 30th or a 200th of such remedies as *Phos.* or *Sil.* might set the economy on the down grade.

From this brief outline of the possibilities of Potency it will be seen that we uphold the use of the high potencies mostly. The question of Potency is the most moot point in all Homoeopathy and even in our ranks today many strict homoeopaths are so-called low-potency men. These follow Hughes and are more pathological in their prescribing. The strict Kentians, almost without exception, are preponderantly high-potency.

The degree of susceptibility of your patient also influences potency selection. Certain persons are over-sensitive (often owing to improper homoeopathic treatment) and they will prove any remedy you give them; they require, therefore, medium-low potencies. Other patients are very sluggish (often owing to much allopathic drugging). These will often take a very high potency to get any action at all, or they may need a low potency repeated every few hours until favourable re-action sets in. A third type of patient is the feeble one where the vital force can easily be overwhelmed. Repetition is the greatest danger here. Acutely sick robust patients will stand repetition of high potencies until favorable reaction commences, although the ideal is the single dose. Children take high potencies particularly well, and in general the very aged require medium potencies except for euthanasia. Some individuals have idiosyncrasies even to homoeopathic potencies of certain substances. Some degree of idiosyncrasy to a remedy must be present or the patient will not be sensitive enough to be cured, but where this is extreme the law of medium potencies should be preferred. Where patients have been habitually poisoned by a crude substance, as a general rule it is not advisable to give that substance in very high potency, it is better to give an antidotal substance high. For instance, patients long dosed with calomel are not relieved by high potencies of *Mercurius*, but may be by *Hepar*. On the other hand exceptions to this occur, as in chronic susceptibility to *Rhus* poisoning. *Rhus tox.* CM may eradicate the tendency. If not, a deeper antipsoric in accordance with the totality of the symptoms is indicated. Certain remedies are noted for their power to restore order after chronic poisoning with crude drugs, as *Natrum mur.* after the misuse of quinine or silver nitrate. The very low potencies, such as the 3 and 6x are very dangerous in the hands of accurate prescribers. This may be mainly due to the customary repetition.

Great care must be taken in potency selection of certain very deep-acting remedies in serious chronic cases. For instance, *Kali carb.* in gout, *Sulph.*, *Sil.*,

Tub., or *Phos.* in tuberculosis; *Psor.* in asthma; and *Arsenicum* and *Lachesis* in many conditions. These remedies should be carried in the 30th potency even by those who give almost entirely the higher degrees.

REPETITION

The single remedy is the third member of the essential homoeopathic trilogy. The reason for this is obvious: only one remedy can be the most similar at any given time with the condition of any given patient. If the physician cannot decide between two remedies he has not got the totality of the symptoms, or the remedies which he has chosen are merely superficially akin to fragments or aspects of the case. Furthermore, the *similimum* is a personality having a rhythm, one might almost say a permeating aura of its own, and in the fleeting instant of its administration it takes complete possession of the patient, thereby buoying up the vital force so that it can carry on the restorative process. To have two or more remedies would be to introduce two separate rhythms, partial and disharmonious factors. Moreover, if more than one remedy be used the doctor cannot know which element was curative, and one source of future guidance is thereby obscured. Lastly, since only one remedy can possibly be proved at a time, so only one can cure at a given moment. Some mongrel homoeopaths when in doubt give mixed prescriptions. This means that they are merely prescribing symptomatically, one remedy for one symptom or organ, and another for another. Each of these, if homoeopathically chosen, may wipe out the fragmentary illness at which it was aimed; but that which is profound, total, and primal, of which all these several symptoms are but manifestations, will remain untouched and simply crop out through other channels as subsequent symptoms. Other half-hearted homoeopaths, and even some with a wide knowledge of the materia medica, but a relatively feeble grasp of the philosophy, alternate remedies. This practice cannot be too strongly condemned, as it seesaws the patient into temporary ups without real progress. Many modern French homoeopaths give a main deep-acting remedy and one or more so-called drainage remedies with it, the chronic remedy in high potency and the drainage remedies in low potency, the idea being that the drainage remedy opens up an outlet for the exodus of the disease. These drainage remedies aim at the production of a discharge or the stimulation of the secretory organs, etc. This is a recent variant and does not appear in Hahnemann, the old masters, or Kent, and the self-styled purists of today do not approve of it.

The subject of the intercurrent remedy may well be mentioned here. Many pure Kentians hold that there is, or should be, no such thing, and that when, after a series of potencies of the same remedy, a new remedy is called for to stir up or develop the case, this is not an intercurrent but at that moment the *similimum*.

There is some division of practice as to whether the single remedy should be given in one or more doses. The high potentists favor the single dose, although two, three, or more doses of a high potency may be given at short intervals—every four, eight, or twelve hours—especially in very acute cases with fever, as the increased metabolism, so to speak, eats up the remedy fast. In such slow diseases as typhoid high potencies may also be repeated close together, but in every instance *it is an absolute rule that when favorable reaction sets in the administration of the remedy must cease*. So long as improvement is visible in the patient himself the remedy should not be repeated. Not only is there no need of "more of a good thing" but a repetition of a remedy which is still acting successfully defeats itself and actually hinders cure. Very occasionally, however, we have found that when a certain potency is aiding somewhat, a higher potency of the same remedy will lift the case to a speedier cure. In this connection it is of interest to mention the theory of double dosage recently promulgated by Gordon of Edinburgh. Gordon gives his remedy in two doses, eight hours apart, the first dose of a lower, and the second of a higher potency of the same remedy. For instance, *Phos.* 200 at bed-time and *Phos.* 1M on rising This has not yet been sufficiently tried out for unqualified acceptance. Some of the masters use a lower potency after a higher one and claim good results. This seems in accord with the order of the progress of disease, from within and above, outward and downward. This has been even less used than the other method and we have no statistics as to whether these cases would have done as well or better on the lower potency originally.

Another method of multiple dosage which almost amounts to divided single doses is that of plussing. "Plussing" means dissolving your dose in a third of a glass of water, taking two teaspoonfuls, throwing away most of the rest, adding water up to the original quantity, stirring and succussing and again taking two teaspoonfuls as the second dose and so on. This raises the potency very slightly between each of the doses, gives somewhat wider range of plane, and is particularly indicated in stubborn and refractory cases. If very low potencies are used in ordinary acute illness, repeated doses are necessary until improvement sets in, in most cases. For instance, a decompensated cardiac case calling for *Crataegus* might need two drops of tincture in water night and morning for a week. Where there is more pathology than vitality this might open the case better than a single high-potency dose of *Crataegus* although this latter might follow later. *Bryonia* 3x should be given as pellets or in water at intervals of one to four hours, according to the pace of the case, in acute cases calling for *Bryonia,* by low-potency men. We would wholeheartedly advocate a single dose of *Bryonia* high, under the same conditions. So much for the administration of the first dose or doses prior to the setting in of a favorable reaction.

Next comes the problem of when to prescribe again. *The rule here is never repeat or change the remedy while the patient himself is improving.* When the improvement has apparently ceased in acute diseases you may need to repeat the same remedy in the same or a higher potency, or, if your remedy was not a *similimum,* you may need another remedy to round out the cure. You must be sure that the cessation of improvement is not due to an emotional, mechanical, or hygienic cause, or merely to the aggravation or outcropping of single symptoms. In chronic work you should wait some time, from three or four days to two or three weeks or more, as the vital force has cycles even on the upward grade, and true curative action must not be interrupted until it is certain that the reactive force is exhausted. Kent admirably stresses this in his injunction to "watch and wait".

As to the interval between repetition of prescriptions, this may vary from a few minutes to a year or more and is entirely dependent on the general amelioration of the patient. When you have had true improvement, and particularly if in chronic cases you have observed the working of Hering's law of cure, sit tight. More cases are bungled by too frequent repetition than by anything else. In this connection it is of course necessary to know which are the long-acting remedies, although we have known of the good effect of *Bryonia* 30, one dose, continuing two years in a chronic condition. Every student should own the little pamphlet by R. Gibson Miller on *The Relationship of Remedies,* which gives approximate duration of action, but the only true guide to the duration of action of any remedy in a given potency on any patient is the cessation of the patient's general sense of well-being. In general, if you are a good prescriber, one dose, single or divided as above, should cope with brief acute diseases, to be followed at the termination of the disease with a chronic to set the economy in order. If a change of remedy is indicated in acute disease there will often be a reversion or return, towards the close of the disease, to the primary remedy.

The subject of the second prescription and of aggravations will be taken up in the next lecture. It remains only to say a word here about the place of *Placebo* in prescribing. A famous doctor said that "*Sac. lac.* is the second best remedy". Patients who understand Homoeopathy deeply may often be content with a single dose at long intervals without *Placebo*, but it is good policy to give even these a single powder of *Placebo* at every visit. Most patients require medicine often, not only so that they feel that something is being done but so that they may have powders for emergencies and it is not only honorable but necessary to give plentiful *Placebo*. It is wise to train the patients to take powders or pellets of *Placebo* which are similar in appearance to the actual remedies, and not to give them the tempting brown, pink, and green blank tablets.

Complicated as these elementary rules sound, they are but the beginning of homoeopathic wisdom. Every student should own and read at least once a year Kent's *Lectures on Homoeopathic Philosophy* and should also be conversant with the writings of Stuart Close, Gibson Miller, John Weir, as well as the *Lectures on Therapeutics* by Dunham and by Joslin and of course, with that keystone of our art—Hahnemann's *Organon*.

PRESCRIBING: AGGRAVATION

Having learned how to select the remedy and the potency, and in how many doses to give it, the next step is to know how to watch your case. The physician must be able to determine whether the remedy given is acting at all, and if so, whether favorably and what prognosis may be expected. He must know how to determine the length of action of his remedy in each individual case; in short, having started the journey to cure, he must be sure that he is in the right train and that he knows when and where to change. Two things help him mainly in these decisions, and both are determined by careful observation based on *seeing* the patient, for what the patient will tell you is often misleading. The first signpost to guide you is the aggravation. A discussion of this is best given in chapters 34 and 35 in Kent's *Lectures on Homoeopathic Philosophy*, from which we have taken much of what follows.

The types of aggravation which may be observed are as follows:

1. A prolonged aggravation with subsequent decline of the patient. This means either that the patient is incurable or that he has been overwhelmed by the tur-

moil ensuing on too high a potency. This usually occurs in cases of marked pathology, yet whose vitality is able to emit symptoms. Under the second prescription we will take up what to do in such exigencies, but the doctor must be sure before resorting to a second prescription that he truly has an aggravation of the first and not the second type.

2. This second type is a long aggravation followed by slow improvement. This means a serious case on the border of incurability but caught just in time.

3. The third type of aggravation is quick, brief, and vigorous, followed by speedy relief of the patient. This type is much to be desired and is a sign that the improvement will be of long duration and that structural changes are in non-vital organs. Abscesses and suppurating glands appear at times in these cases as part of the aggravation. This is a good sign and should not be interfered with.

4. The fourth type is where there is practically no observable aggravation and yet the patient recovers steadily. This is ideal and shows that there is no great organic disease and that the potency chosen exactly fits the case, especially if during recovery the symptoms follow Hering's laws, which will be discussed later.

5. The fifth type is where brief amelioration comes first and aggravation afterwards. This means either that your remedy was only palliative and did not touch the true constitutional state of the patient, or else that the patient is incurable, or else that some deeper miasmatic remedy is needed, like a mordant to enable the indicated remedy (or dye, to follow out our simile) to take hold. For example, a *Silica* case of ours would be markedly ameliorated for a week or ten days and then slip back, nor did a change of potency hold longer; however, *Tuberculinum* took hold and kept it, and since then other remedies hold.

6. Another type of aggravation is where the symptoms developed turn out to be a proving of your rem-

edy. This may be due to an idiosyncrasy to the particular drug on the part of your patient, or the patient may be an over-sensitive who proves everything given him. These patients need the medium-low potencies and are often incurable.

7. Another apparent form of aggravation is where new symptoms appear after the administration of a remedy. This suggests that the prescription was incorrect, and will be dealt with under the second prescription.

8. There is a type of aggravation in which the individual symptoms stand out more clearly while the patient himself feels better. This is often followed by old symptoms reappearing in the reverse order of their coming. (See Hering's laws of cure.) This is highly favorable. The physician must note the direction of the appearing symptoms. If they go wrongly, *i.e.*, from without inward, it is dangerous; if from within outward it is favorable.

Another variant, which is without actual aggravation, is too short a relief of symptoms, without any special aggravation. This is very similar to the fifth, and causes the physician to cast about for a miasmatic remedy.

Sometimes there is a full-time amelioration of symptoms without any special relief to the patient himself. This shows a case that is only open to palliation, the vital force cannot make the grade of cure.

An unnecessarily severe aggravation is caused by too high or too low a potency. A well-chosen potency will give, as above, either no aggravation or a quick short one. Too prolonged an aggravation may be caused by giving too low a potency or by repeating. In the aggravations after high potencies such as CM, in curable cases, the patient feels distinctly better even during the aggravation, as it is the characteristic symptoms and not the disease or the patient which are aggravated.

A very feeble vitality may not be able to throw out

an aggravation, and such must be given a single dose of a really high potency and watched for the minutest signs. On the other hand, a strong vitality may have marked tissue changes which will produce a violent aggravation; so that the physician must bear in mind the two factors, the vitality of the whole and the pathological changes, and balance these carefully in his choice of potency.

If there is no aggravation in cases of vigorous vitality, it is probable that your remedy was only partially similar. (The ideal cases of recovery without perceptible aggravation are usually not those with especially marked vitality.) In acute diseases an amelioration without a slight initial aggravation often means that your remedy is not deep enough and another dose of it will probably be needed.

THE SECOND PRESCRIPTION

Kent defines the second prescription as "the one after one that has acted." This means that a bungling prescriber may have given four or five remedies and that the sixth, if it really takes hold, should be classed as the first prescription. Granted that according to the above observations on aggravation your remedy was well-chosen and has acted, *let it alone*. "Watch and wait." Before making any second prescription *re-study the case*. According to Kent there are three possibilities for the second prescription, either *repetition, antidoting, or complementing*.

The prime indication for the second prescription which is a *repetition* is the return of the original symptoms of the patient. The patient has been better, with or without aggravation, and then he tells you, and you observe, that the original symptoms have reappeared, whether identical, less severe, or more severe than at first. This calls for repetition in the same potency, after you are sure they have returned to stay. It should here be added that if the patient returns telling you that his general sense of well-being has come to a standstill, but his original symptoms have not yet returned, you should wait, as often improvement goes in cycles, and the good work will begin again of itself. Even if he tells you that he himself feels worse, wait and watch for return of the original symptoms before repeating. Moreover, even if the symptoms change, but the patient feels and seems still improved, do not change your remedy. It would be chasing will-o'-the-wisps to do so and you would ruin your case. While well-being increases, wait; when it comes to standstill, wait. If the general state is worse and the symptoms have changed then consider a new second prescription as follows:

The prime indication for a change of remedy in the second prescription is where new symptoms crop up after your first prescription, without amelioration in the general well-being of the patient, and remain. This means the first prescription was unfavorable and you must antidote it. The selection of this antidotal second prescription is based on the original symptoms plus the new symptoms, with more emphasis on the new ones. This second prescription, then, should wipe out the new symptoms and modify the old.

The prime indication for a change to a complementary remedy is where your first prescription, especially in acute disease or if it was not a deep-acting remedy, does not seem to have fathomed the case. Here a complementary remedy will take deeper hold on the life. For instance, in an acute throat *Belladonna* may be the *similimum,* but, after the acute attack has passed, a chaser may be needed to prevent recurrence, to eradicate predisposition, and, if the symptoms agree, your second prescription would be the chronic complement of *Belladonna,* which is *Calcarea.*

There is another indication, which goes deep into the philosophy, for a change of remedy in your second prescription. This is likely to be a remedy for a different miasmatic group and it entails a change in the plan of treatment, consequent to the cropping up of a different miasm after the clearing away by the first prescription of the miasm which was at first on top of the case.

This subject of the second prescription was to me the most difficult Homoeopathy. Every beginner should read and re-read his Kent's *Philosophy,* re-study his cases, and above all "watch and wait."

REMEDY RELATIONSHIPS

The subject of the relationship of remedies is one of the most fascinating in Homoeopathy, and many aspects of it have not been developed in the literature. Long before Hahnemann, Paracelsus wrote much on the doctrine of signatures, and the old herbalists determined the uses of their remedies partly from those suggested signs. A vast amount of work on the relationship of remedies to each other, rather than to symptoms, has been done by such men as Boenninghausen, Hering, Clarke, Gibson Miller, the Allens, Kent, Guernsey, and Lippe. Most of this work has been along one main line, that of *complementary* remedies, in other words, those remedies which carry on or complete most successfully the action of other given remedies. Certain disparities exist in the lists of the above men, and the lists in the original should be studied by the student. The best sources for this are: Gibson Miller's little pamphlet, *The Relationship of Remedies*, printed in London but obtainable from Boericke and Tafel in Philadelphia (no homoeopathic practitioner should be without one; when your case has repertorized out to three or four remedies and it seems evident that no *similimum* will unravel the whole condition, and at the moment it is impossible to decide which of two to give first, Miller's tables will often indicate that one follows the other to better advantage than *vice versa*); the fourth volume of Clarke's *Dictionary*, the *Clinical Repertory*, which contains the same type of tables and material on a greater number of remedies, although we feel that Gibson Miller has pruned wisely; and the very suggestive grouping of remedies by Teste, in his *Materia Medica* (unfortunately he does not explain how he arrived at his groupings).

There are several classes of complementary relationships. A word of explanation about the practical application of each is in order: a plain complementary remedy, such as those listed immediately below, is related by symptomatology; and sometimes, as in the case of *Ars.-Phos.*, by occurrence in nature; and sometimes by constituents, e.g., *Badiaga-Iodum*. In explanation of this type of complementary remedy it may be said that ideally "one remedy, one dose" should cure, but most cases are so mixed, so confused by miasms, drugging, etc., that one must tack against the wind, using more than one remedy. Some of the main complementary relationships of this type are as follows:

Ant. tart.-Ip.	*Cham.-Mag. carb.*	*Nat. sulph.-Thuja*
Apis-Nat. mur.	*China-Ferrum*	*Op.-Plb.*
Arg. nit.-Nat. mur.	*Con.-Bar. mur.*	*Petr.-Sep.*
Ars.-Phos.	*Cupr.-Calc.*	*Phos.-Carbo veg., Ars.*
Bar. carb.-Dulc.	*Iod.-Lyc.*	*Puls.-Kali sulph.*
Berb. vulg.-Lyc.	*Lach.-Lyc., Nit. ac.*	*Sab.-Thuja*
Bry.-Rhus	*Med.-Sulph.*	*Stan.-Puls.*
Calc.*-Rhus	*Mez.-Merc.*	

*For *Bell.* see under acute and chronic.

A more specialized class of complementary remedies is the *acute* complements of chronic remedies or the *chronic* complements of acute remedies, according to whether your patient is first seen as an acute or a chronic case. For instance, an acute *Bell.* throat, to prevent recurrence and finish off the case, may need the chronic complement, *Calcarea;* or a chronic *Natrum mur.* case may develop an acute cold which will call for its acute complement, *Bryonia.* One of the confusing points is that a chronic remedy may have more than one acute complement; for example, *Natrum mur.* has *Bryonia, Ignatia,* and *Apis; Lyc.* has *Rhus, Chel.,* and *Puls.,* and sometimes *Iod.* Some of the best known examples, putting the acutes first, are:

Acon.-Sulph.	*Coloc.-Staph.*
Ars.-Thuja	*Hepar-Sil.*
Bac.-Calc. phos.	*Nux vom.-Sep.*
Bell.-Calc.	*Puls.-Sil.*
Bry.-Alum., Nat. mur.	

The third type of complementary remedies is one on which the least work has been done, most of the data being found sprinkled around in Kent's *Materia Medica.* These are remedies *in series.* For instance, *Calc.-Lyc.-Sulph.* (it will be noted that all three of these are chronic remedies; they must be used in this order and not the opposite one); *Ign.-Nat. mur.-Sepia; Puls.-Sil.-Fluor. ac.; Ars.-Thuja-Tarent.; All. cep.-Phos.-Sulph.; Acon.-Spongia-Hepar;* and many others.

Of course only a few examples from among those listed in the suggested study books have been given here. The student will notice that for the most part the nosodes have been omitted; also the tissue salts; moreover certain notable remedies, like *Kali carb.,* for which many complements have been suggested but none seems wholly satisfactory.

In the above sources certain remedies are listed as *incompatible*. This means not only that these remedies are not given together by the true Hahnemannian homoeopath, but it means that they must not follow each other without an intervening remedy or considerable time. Some of these are as follows:

Acon.-Acet. ac.	*Ign.-Coff., Nux, Tab.*
Amm. carb.-Lach.	*Lach.-Dulc., Psor.*
Apis-Rhus	*Led.-Chin.*
Aur. mur. natr.-	*Lyc.* after *Sulph.*
Coffea	
Bell.-Dulc.	*Merc.-Sil.,* and *before Bar.*
Calc. after *Kali bi.*	*carb.* or *Sulph.*
or *Nit. ac.*	*Phos.-Caust.*
Caust.-Phos.	*Psor.-Sep.*
Cham.-Nux, Zinc.	*Rhus-Apis*
Cocc.-Coff.	*Sep.-Lach.*
Ferrum after *Dig.*	

The subject of *remedy analogues* in the animal, vegetable, and mineral kingdoms has been but little studied and offers a fruitful field. (Some hold that theoretically there should be a remedy in each of the three kingdoms for every ill.) Examples are: *Ignatia* is the vegetable analogue of *Natrummur.;* and *Phytolacca* of *Mercury*.

The relationships of remedies according to their chemical constituents is a highly interesting and all too undeveloped subject. It illuminates relationships, as for instance, *Pulsatilla* contains *Kali sulph.; Bell.* has much *Mag. phos.;* and *Allium cepa* and *Lyc.* contain *Sulph.* Quantitative chemical analyses should be done on all our vegetable remedies. Among the animal remedies, *Badiaga* and *Spongia* contain *Iodine*.

The botanical relationships of the vegetable remedies are very suggestive. These are to be found in Clarke's *Clinical Repertory*. The student would do well to familiarise himself with the better known remedies in this group, a few of which are given below:

Loganiaceae:
  Brucea
  Curare
  Gels.
  Hoang nan
  Ign.
  Nux
  Spig.
  Upas
Ranunculaceae:
  Adonis
  Clem.
  Hepatica
  Hydrastis
  Puls.
  Ran. bulb.
  Ran. scel.
  Aconites
  Actea rac.
    (Cimic.)

Actea spic.
Aquil. vulg.
Caltha pal.
Hellebores
Staph.
Poeonia
Rubiaceae:
  Cahinca
  Coff.
  Mitchella
  China
  Ip.
  Galium
  Rubia tinct.
Solanaceae:
  Bell.
  Caps.
  Duboisin
  Daturas

Dulc.
Hyos.
Lycopersicum
  (tomato)
Mandragora
Pichi
Solanums
  (potato, etc.)
Stram.
Tab.
Berberidaceae:
  Berb.
  Caul.
  Podo.
Melanthaceae:
  Colch.
  Helonias
  Sabad.
  Verat.
  Yucca

Some of the therapeutic snags in connection with the relationship of remedies will be taken up in a later lecture on the dangers of homoeopathic prescribing.

PATHOLOGICAL PRESCRIBING

Few things are more stimulating than to have our own pet prejudices successfully attacked. One of the fundamental principles which is drilled into every good Kentian homoeopathic student is that one must not prescribe pathologically. For the allopathic convert to adopt this point of view is one of the most difficult obstacles to the acquiring of Homoeopathy. By dint of much drilling it finally becomes ingrained. We realize that it is the patient and his individual reaction to the so-called disease who must be prescribed for. We realize that pathology is an ultimate, an exteriorization, a protective out-throwing, or excrescence, or discharge on the part of the organism. Our tendency is, then, to throw pathology overboard and to disregard both symptoms and organic facts which we class under that head. If we do not take great care we find that we are not succeeding as we should, that we are giving remedies on functional symptoms only, which remedies do not have it in their power to produce, and so cure, the given pathology. We may stop a hemorrhage from a fibroid uterus with a remedy which has not the ability to produce fibroids in its nature. This will be suppression. We may relieve pain and fever in a case of pleuritic exudate with a lightweight remedy, but we will not cause resorption of this exudate by any such superficial treatment. So, little by little, our own experience, as well as that of many master prescribers, will bring it home to us that *pathology is to be considered in prescribing*, not as the sole basis, but as an important factor in the totality of the symptoms. We come to see that the pathology also reveals the patient. A tendency to polypi is a valuable symptom. We must know our pathology in all cases, even those which have abundant non-pathological symptoms, for diagnostic purposes, to satisfy the patient, to govern our prognosis, and especially to determine our choice of potency and remedy. Where there is marked organic change a safe rule is to give the lower potencies, although often in a vital person a high potency, if the true *similimum*, will cause great amelioration of the patient and drive the disease out faster into or through the pathology. This may alarm or inconvenience the patient, but the true homoeopath will understand and will explain it to the patient and his family. It will influence the choice of our remedy in that it will make us give a drug big enough to cope with the situation. It will teach us when the case is incurable, and warn us away from giving too high a potency, thereby causing a severe aggravation from which the economy cannot rally. It will show us in incurable and precarious cases of chronic disease, or even in such acute ones as early tuberculosis, when we must eschew the true *similimum* and give a palliative remedy or a less deep-acting remedy as a preparative for the true *similimum*. In cases, and there are not so many, when the alert homoeopath cannot find subjective symptoms or modalities he must resort to prescribing on pathology.

Often pathology also is a general, for Kent himself tells us that a condition appearing in three or more particulars ranks as a general. Such symptoms as excessive discharges, which Dr. Boger classes in his

General Analysis under "moistness," may also lead us to the true inner nature of the patient.

There is another type of pathology which Dr. G. B. Stearns classes as objective symptoms—in other words, pathology visible to the eye. This may not mean organic tissue change which is unalterable, and includes such rewarding details as redness of the orifices, fissures, herpes, eruptions, skin discolorations, warts, moles, peculiarities of hair, nails, etc. In children, especially, these objective symptoms are often our best guide.

It behooves us, therefore, even the strictest Hahnemannians among us, to give the pathological symptom its due!

THE PROBLEM OF SUPPRESSION

A patient said to me recently, "Where can I find literature showing the dangers of suppression? My daughter wants to put ointment on her baby's scalp eczema and won't believe me when I tell her it is perilous to do so." This made me search the literature which I found very meagre. Therefore this attempt to state the problem, the discussion of which in this body should be of real importance.

First, let us define the term: by suppression is meant that a disease manifestation is caused to disappear before the disease itself is cured.

The subject of suppression seems one of the most important from the homoeopathic point of view, but one of the least familiar to the ordinary medical mind. In regular medicine we are continually meeting with examples of suppression; indeed, from our point of view, all of usual medicine which is not unconscious Homoeopathy is suppressive. There are various types of suppression.

1. Suppressions accidental or natural and not due to medication of any kind, such as suppression of strong emotion due to the unnatural exigencies of our collective living. These are more or less conscious suppressions, although the seriousness of their results is not usually known and the individual takes great pride and credit in thrusting down these emotions.

There is a second kind of accidental suppression which comes from great mental shocks such as mortification or grief.

A third type of natural suppression is in the physical realm, such as where the menses are checked by injudicious bathing, or the lochia stopped after labor by catching cold, or milk suppressed, or perspiration suddenly inhibited by chilling.

Then there is also a type of suppression of one disease by another, which is so frequently spoken of in the *Organon*. This may take the form of an acute disease being held in abeyance by another acute one until the "cure" of the second; or it may be an acute disease suspending a chronic until the acute course is run. The reverse of this, where a chronic disease holding sway gives a partial or full measure of immunity against acute disease, could really be classed as suppression although it is more usually thought of as immunity.

2. A second type of suppression most frequent in regular medicine nowadays is suppressions by local applications. This enters into many fields. For instance, coryzas and sinus troubles are suppressed by local applications of argyrol, iodine, and other substances; leucorrheal and gonorrheal discharges by injection of mercurochrome, protargol and permanganate; eruptions, from such acute ones as scabies and impetigo through to the chronic ones such as eczema and psoriasis, by zinc or sulphur preparations, ammoniated mercury, and many others. The rashes due to the exanthems, which may also be classed under natural suppression in some instances, may be driven in by the unwise use of cold packs. Other secretions, such as foot-sweat, are often suppressed by foot powder; conjunctival pus by silver salts; ulcers by various local dressings; and warts by trichloracetic acid or electrical means. We have further the local suppression of many conditions by the different lamps, violet-ray therapy, etc.

Hemorrhages are suppressed by local astringents,

such as tannic acid, or by local coagulants such as thromboplastin, or by X-ray. (They may also be suppressed by general medication such as calcium lactate and gelatin.) This brings up the question as to whether a homoeopathic drug such as *Ceanothus americanus* should be classed as suppressive or curative.

3. Now we come to conditions suppressed by current internal medication: for instance, malaria, which, if not of the quinine type, is simply suppressed by the massive routine quinine dosage, often resulting in recurrent neuralgia; acute rheumatic fever where the patient is overpowered with salicylates, leading to suppression of joint symptoms and the inroads of the disease on the heart; epilepsy and choreas are often driven to cover by saturation with sedatives; and heart disease masked by digitalis.

4. Disease is all too frequently suppressed by surgery: the removal of growths, benign or malign, polypi, tonsils, appendices, varicosities, hemorrhoids, fistulae, and bone hypertrophies such as turbinates. The trouble here is that modern medicine seeks to remove pathology rather than cure the underlying causes, not realizing that the ultimates of disease are benign attempts at exteriorization, at protective localizations.

5. Most insidious of all are the suppressions by vaccine injections, which are now so prevalent that a child may take seven or eight different kinds in a year. I know a family of seven children of a well-known allopathic physician who were given in one year cold vaccines, diphtheria, scarlet fever, whooping cough, typhoid, paratyphoid, and smallpox, and two of the seven were also given hayfever pollen inoculations.

6. There is the whole question of the old suppressions of syphilis by arsenical and mercurial treatment, which many doctors, even of the regular school, feel tends to develop later grave nervous tertiaries as well as saddling the patients with drug results.

7. There is another aspect of suppression, that of the suppression of individual symptoms, and this may be

done quite as effectively by the use of homoeopathic remedies as by old-school drugs. Never forget that to palliate a curable case is suppression. It will involve you in continual change of remedies, a sort of "puss in the corner" with the symptoms. It will mask the true fundamental picture of the disease and complicate it to the point where it will be incurable. The degree to which this is done by the general run of homoeopathic practitioners and by exuberant self-medicating laymen is not realized and is appalling.

I need not go into the bad results of these different kinds of suppression, you have all seen them. They include asthma, convulsions, paralysis, insanity, tuberculosis, and deep diseases of the vital organs. Last year Dr. Stearns gave a paper on *Prodromal Symptoms and Their Importance in Prescribing*. This paper of mine should be entitled *Prodromal or Prior Suppressions, Their Importance in Prescribing*. In every case we must *"cherchez"* not *"la femme"* but *"la suppression."* Shall we prescribe for the symptoms before the suppression took place? Shall we use the form of suppression as a symptom in our totality? Shall we prescribe mainly for the present post-suppressive syndrome? We must remember that suppression in any of its forms drives diseases in, masks symptoms, makes protean changes in the form of the disease and blocks the natural exit of the disease. Always leave the golden bridge of your pathological ultimates, as by that route only can the disease return to cure. Disease is the Minotaur in the Labyrinth. Theseus, the symptom, must find his way back and out of the Labyrinth. Do not cut his cord!

THE MANAGEMENT OF THE
HOMOEOPATHIC PATIENT

Where do we get our *patients* to manage? Either referred from patients we have helped, or from other homoeopathic doctors, or the homoeopathic pharmacy (if we are lucky enough to live where there is one), or acquaintances of friends who are discouraged with usual medicine.

Our duty to them as homoeopaths is manifold:

First in importance, is to *pick the right remedy* and to remove obstacles to cures.

To stop harmful practices and give placebo if needed to keep them from taking other things.

To give them enough understanding of homeopathic philosophy to cooperate in their cure.

To institute proper diet, hygiene, protection, and state of mind.

Second, to win the patient's confidence by what *you* are—by your profound humanity, by your ability to see them as they could be, *whole*.

By your painstaking thoroughness in questioning and in examination.

By your attitude toward science, having tests when these are harmless and diagnostically helpful.

Many of the most truly homoeopathic doctors object to this on the grounds that thay do not *need laboratory tests,* nor a *diagnosis* for *cure.* Often they do *not* need it for *symptom removal;* in functional cases, not even for cure. But modern patients in my experience are too medicine-conscious, through magazines if nothing else, and class you as unscientific and lose respect for you if you disregard all this. Moreover your actual prescribing will be improved if you know the pathological tendencies—and conditions.

The second act of our homoeopathic drama is, to me, far more dfficult: the determination of when another remedy is needed. Many of the most satisfactory homoeopathically trained patients can be allowed to ride on a remedy which is helping until they themselves tell you they need another boost. But many will feel neglected and must be seen daily even when you know you will not change the remedy. If you have a competent nurse on the case, who notes symptoms well, she can often tell whether you are really needed and help you convince the family if you are not. On the other hand a nervous or inept nurse needs the reassurance of your frequent presence. (Someday I'd like to write a parody of Seton-Thompson's book and title it: *Wild Nurses I Have Known!)* It takes one's utmost self-control, tact, and patience to deal with families; to keep the delicate balance between hope and fear—in critical cases—so that their forces are not exhausted yet they are somewhat prepared for possible bad outcome.

One of the conventional questions in case management is always "Shall the doctor tell the patients if they have a serious or fatal disease?" A wise man once said, "When it is time for them to know, they will know and tell *you.* After that you can discuss it with them." But for one's own protection, if one is sure of the diagnosis, a near relative must be told. Yet untold harm is done by doctors making brutal statements both of diagnosis and prognosis. Human resilience is incredible.

I was called recently—emergency—to a woman of

65 in a tonic convulsion, blue with rolling eyes, stertorous breathing, and cold sweat. Not incontinent. She had never had such an attack. The family thought she was dying. Her pupils reacted to light and were equal, there was no Babinski. They were lamenting as though she were not there, but I could see in her eyes that she understood. The thumbs were drawn in. *Cupr.* followed by *Opium* 1M brought her around in an hour or so and that afternoon she wanted to get up and do her washing!

Many suggestible patients are convinced that they have diseases or will have them which they definitely have *not*. No amount of reassurance avails with some, but a simple statement that "You just haven't the symptoms of that," with a little smile, will do wonders. (Never tell such a one what the symptoms *are*, though!)

To go back a moment to another reason why homoeopaths need diagnosis: I lost a delightful family as patients because I kept my diagnosis to myself. A cocky boy of 11 returned from boarding school where they had mumps, and his mother 'phoned me he had it and to come and see him. "But you aren't swollen or sore in the mumps gland—the parotid." "Oh, I have it, though," said he. He was a very *Phosphorus* type of child. He had cervical adenitis. I had worried about the possibility of tuberculosis with him and built him up with remedies. I had actually given him *Tub. bov.* 1M, but had not told the mother, who was very apprehensive, lest I scare her, knowing I could cope with the condition. She thought he didn't get well quick enough for mumps, called another doctor who diagnosed tubercular glands, and I lost the family. Since then I write a letter to myself containing the diagnosis and *post* it to myself and keep it on file unopened in such cases!

The most difficult cases to manage are the new patients who don't yet understand what they must *not* do: that they must *not* suppress again an eruption or dis-

75

charge that the homoeopath has been trying to bring out again. Always warn your patients with suppressions in their histories, if a rash or discharge reoccurs, to do *nothing* and let you know.

Aggravations are not so hard to handle if you warn patients. Tell them that they may occur and that it will be a good sign if they do.

Another problem is the veteran patient with access to homoeopathic remedies. Give out-of-towners or in accessibles with children cases of remedies by all means, but *numbered,* not named, and have them 'phone you which to give. Be sure there are various bottles of placebo under different names. But even then they will vex you: In one kit I gave, No. 18 is *Sepia.* My patient found it so effective for her state of mind that she got to taking it on her own! Maybe we should call in the cases for revision and change the signals!

One of the worst problems is when the patient has a disease considered fatal, for which there is the prescribed treatment which at least prolongs life, or where the disease is *rare* and there are no data of treatment by pure Homoeopathy in large series of cases. For instance I have a case of myologenous leukemia in a man of 42. X-ray therapy of the spleen is *de riguer.* He and his friends would not consider omitting it. Nor do I consider myself justified in urging it, as I would the omission of quinine in malaria, sulfa drugs in pneumonia, etc. I *believe* Homoeopathy can help *this* case, for the man comes out clearly to a remedy *(Phosphorus)* and the case has had suppression enough (psoriasis, sinus, piles, etc.) to give any fatal trouble. *But* am I justified in trying to battle for *Phosphorus* alone? He has improved on it, although his blood count rises periodically. He is stronger and work more than he should. His post-nasal drip has returned, and an eruption. He then got a sore throat away from New York and a doctor friend gave him 150 grains of sulfadiazine. He returned looking ghastly. There is one case surely in which the diagnosis is like a millstone around the neck!

One danger of the homoeopathic doctor is to be a sphinx, another to be euphoric. It takes balance, character, firmness, and faith and untiring industry to be even a decent homoeopath.

No paper, however brief, on homoeopathic case management should go without comment on what you may let the patient do while the remedy is working; calendula ointment, echinacea succus, oil of lavender, pinus pumilio salves, hydrotherapy, mullein oil, plantago oil, arnica cerate, postural drainings in ears, normal salt solution as a cathartic and in beginning migraines.

As to the real essence of remedy management, you can read your Kent on *The Second Prescription* and the types of aggravations. Philosophy can be learned from books, but I have yet to see a book or hear a course in medical schools on the thousand and one things that make a doctor a great success in private practice and with patients.

In the end, as in all things, the effective management of the patients is dependent on how one manages oneself, for we do not teach or learn by what is said but from what we feel and sense and know and are.

PROBLEMS CONFRONTING ONE WHEN FIRST ATTEMPTING TO PRESCRIBE HOMOEOPATHICALLY

Before discussing the problems of actual homoeopathic practice let me show you some of the difficulties in the ordinary practice of medicine which led me to an interest in Homoeopathy. When I was a student at Columbia Medical School, "P & S" as we called it, in the war time, I was much disappointed at the paucity of therapeutic information. There was pathology and bacteriology galore, and fascinating drill in diagnosis, but being a woman and therefore a practical soul (I see some of you smiling at women you have met), I hankered after means of cure. Most of what we were taught in therapeutics was hygiene, nursing procedures, diet, hydrotherapy, etc. A large proportion of my class who had intended to go into general medicine took up surgery or the specialties, because in those fields there was something definite to do for the patients. From medical school I went to Bellevue Hospital for two years' rotating internship, and there again I met the prevailing therapeutic nihilism. Our chief of service was a wizard at diagnosis, but I always felt that an autopsy was fully as acceptable to him as a cure, and much more frequent. One class of patients in the hospital particularly distressed me, those who had abundant subjective symptoms and on whom the diagnostic and laboratory pronouncement was, "There is nothing wrong with you." I remember one saying, "Well, doctor, I may be perfectly well, but *I* know I am sick." And then there were the chronics, not only those with marked pathology, but life-long sufferers from "indigestion" or migraine, who had been passed around from doctor to doctor with nothing but temporary relief. Two other problems puzzled me particularly in those days besides the apparently functional cases and the chronics. One of these was the patient with a classically recognizable disease who did not respond to the usual "specific" treatment for that disease. For instance, a young sailor with a severe malaria which no amount of quinine influenced in the least, to the consternation of all the visiting physicians. (He needed *Eup. perf.*, not *Chin.*) The other matter which set me thinking was the wide variety of types of a single disease. I used to wonder why the pneumonia in the second bed who was such a strapping specimen, and had come down suddenly at midnight on the date of admission, was in such mortal terror of dying by noon the next day (which I may add, he did, to the surprise of all of us); and why the besotted looking fellow in the next bed lay on the affected side with his hand under his chest, motionless, gulping two or three glasses of water at long intervals, complaining of the light and snapping your head off when spoken to; and why the pneumonia on the other side of the ward thrashed about so incessantly, especially in the evening, calling for cold milk. Now I know that although these three had the same disease and received the same treatment, they would have responded to three different remedies, *Aconite, Bryonia,* and *Rhus tox.* But that is getting ahead of our story. My puzzles, then, in my training, were the apparently functional cases, the chronics, the patients who did not respond to the classical treatment of a clearly marked disease, and the varied types classified and treated according to one diagnosis.

Dr. Underhill has told you most graphically and humorously how *he* was led into Homoeopathy, so I will omit my initiation except to say that after working at the *Allgemeine Krankenhaus* in Vienna in the usual way, I was apprenticed for nine months to a homoeopathic physician in Geneva, where I studied, literally, from 12 to 16 hours a day.

Before he was willing to take me as a pupil he gave me a stiff examination in ordinary medicine, including anatomy, fractures, surgical diagnosis, pathology, bacteriology, and chemistry, and gave me slides to diagnose under the microscope, etc. He then asked me certain questions as to what I thought life was about, why I went into the practice of medicine, what were the chief duties of a physician and so on. These questions perplexed me, as I did not then understand their bearing on the philosophy of Homoeopathy. He then put to me a leading question to see if I already had any background of Homoeopathy. It was, "What do homoeopaths give for rheumatism?" Having read somewhat in homoeopathic liteature I answered that homoeopaths do not give a remedy for rheumatism or for any disease name or diagnosis (although, of course, certain remedies are more frequently indicated in rheumatic conditions). They give a remedy on the symptoms of the patient who has the disease, in other words, on the reaction of the individual in question to any given disease entity. This defines one of the fundamental differences between the homoeopathic approach and regular medicine.

Until the physician's mind has encompassed the differences between the viewpoints of ordinary medical training and Homoeopathy, he cannot even begin to prescribe homoeopathically. Let me enumerate, for clarity, wherein these differences lie. First, as above mentioned, he must grasp the principle of *individualization*. Modern medicine lays a good foundation for this through its interest in endocrinology and psychiatry, but except for obvious glandular imbalances, it offers, as yet, no therapy commensurate with the refinements of differentiation. What does individualization mean to the homoeopath and how does he arrive at it? It involves a subsidiary new method of casetaking. After you have your classical history, elicited largely by asking questions, you can often make a diagnosis but rarely a homoeopathic prescription. For the latter you need to know the *mental* state of your patient, and what the homoeopaths call his *"generals,"* which mean the things which apply to the patient as a whole—his reaction to heat and cold, wet and dry weather, and storms, motion, position, food, etc. You need to know how these same factors affect the specific complaints of your patient, in other words, the *modalities* of his particular disease symptoms— whether his headache is better from hot or cold applications, from motion or rest, from lying or walking, from pressure, or food, and at what time of day it is worse. ("Modalities," in other words, mean aggravations or ameliorations of specific symptoms, just as "Generals" mean aggravations and ameliorations of the patient as a whole.) There is a fourth type of thing that you must know about your patient in order to prescribe homoeopathically and that is his rare, peculiar, or characteristic *particular* symptoms. These often appear trivial idiosyncrasies to the patient, things that he has always had, or that no doctor to whom he has told them has ever been interested in. These often serve as *keynotes* to guide you to a remedy. But of what use is all this additional information about your patient? How does this picture of his personality aid you? You have individualized, but of what use is such differentiation, if you have only a standard treatment for the condition that you have diagnosed?

This brings us to the second great difference between Homoeopathy and regular medicine. The law on which Homoeopathy is based, or, if you prefer, the hypothesis, is to be found in the statement of Hippocrates, "*similia similibus curentur*," which Hahnemann revived and amplified. Dr. Stearns has told you how Hahnemann came to apply this law and made the first so-called "proving" of quinine. A "proving," in the homoeopathic sense, is experimenting with a drug in minute doses on relatively healthy human being. The record of symptoms so produced, on a large number of provers of different ages and sexes, constitutes the basis of our homoeopathic matera medica. The object of proving a drug is to delineate the drug personality. Each of our remedies is to us a living individual, they are like friends whom one recognizes whenever seen, not only by their grand characteristics but also by their mannerisms and tricks. We now have, on the one hand, the drug personalities, and on the other, the picture of our patient in his present state. It follows, if like cures like, that we must match pictures and fit the personality of a drug to our patient, administer it, and watch the results. After one has grasped this ingenious theory and learned to put it into practice, it remains only to see it work. I, for one, being a natural sceptic, was slow to believe the evidence of my senses. Could the astonishing improvements and cures have been coincidence or suggestion, or faulty diagnosis? There are certain controls which one can use. Put the patient on the proper regimen, including diet, etc., and see what that alone does for your condition. Then give *Placebo*, with your best manner. In my experience, in nine cases out of ten the patient will report no progress. When they are discouraged by this unsuccessful first prescription, give them the remedy you have chosen, the *similimum*. If you feel reasonably certain that the drug picture fits your patient, and you have the *similimum*, in most cases you will see a swift and beautiful result. But these are not the only possible methods of control. There are laws of remedy action which are contrary to anything you could expect in an untreated case. When you see these, you know that your remedy is taking hold. They were formulated by Constantine Hering, one of the pioneers of Homoeopathy in this country, and are as follows: The curative remedy acts *from within outward, from above downward,* and *in the reverse order of the symptoms.* Take as an illustration a case of rheumatic fever in which, after the customary salicylate dosing, the joints appear to have cleared up but a heart condition develops. Give such a patient the similar remedy and he will complain that his joints are worse again, but *he himself* feels better and you find that his heart is clearing up. You explain to him that the remedy is working *from within outward;* the more vital organ, the heart, is getting well first, and the peripheral organs, the joints, are again involved. Give him nothing but *Placebo.* Shortly he will tell you that his shoulders and wrists are clearing up, but that the pain is now in his knees or ankles. Again you see the law of cure in action, *from above downward,* and you wait. You observe that his symptoms are disappearing *in the reverse order of their appearance,* the heart condition, which came last, going first. If you trust your remedy under these conditions, your patient will make a real recovery without the annoying recurrences. (If, on the contrary, you found that the joints in the lower extremities cleared up and those of the upper extremities became involved, you would know you were on the wrong track and had not found the *similimum.*)

One of the knottiest problems for the beginner is the different concept of pathology and bacteriology. Homoeopaths accept the facts of these branches of medicine. The difference lies in the interpretation. Pathology is an end result of some morbid process. The homoeopath is not nearly as interested in the diseased tonsil, the hemorrhoid, the ovarian cyst, the cancer, the tapeworm, or the psoriasis, as he is in the constitutional dyscrasia behind these. He is not eager to remove the ultimates of disease at once, but rather to cure the underlying cause. In the course of this cure the ultimate will often disappear, as in the case of diseased cervical glands or fibroids. If not, it can be removed when it has become merely a foreign body, and when the constitution is so changed that it will not ultimate itself in further pathology in a more deep-seated organ. Similarly one is taught to consider that bacteria cause disease. The homoeopath is more interested in the individual's susceptibility, than in the bacteria themselves. Instead of poisoning the malarial plasmodia with quinine or the syphilitic spirochaetae with salvarsan, the homoeopath prefers to stimulate the body to make itself uninhabitable for these organisms, and he does this by means of the similar remedy. To give another instance, instead of killing off head lice with delphinium and leaving the patient susceptible to further invasions, the homoeopath gives a chronic constitutional remedy which removes the susceptibility, and the lice seek better pasturage.

A fourth stumbling block for the medical mind is the question of suppression. Discharges and eruptions are ordinarily classed with pathology as something to be gotten rid of by local measures. We are taught to use argyrol in coryzas, to paint cervices with mercurochrome in leucorrhoea, to stop a gonorrheal discharge with protargol or penicillin, to check a diarrhea with opium or bismuth, to clear up skin eruptions with ammoniated mercury or sulphur ointment or other applications. The homoeopath holds that this is suppression, and not cure, that these outward manifestations are not primarily local but an expression of deep disease, the body trying to throw off impurities. They have watched the incidence of more deep-seated troubles following such "suppression." The chronic constitutional homoeopathic remedy given to a case which has been so treated will often bring back the original eruption or discharge, with concomitant relief of recent grave symptoms and ultimate clearing up from *within* of the original discharge or eruption. Let me illustrate with a case from my practice recently. A woman of 45 came to me for suicidal depression, for which she could give no emotional cause. She dated her mental symptoms definitely from the time when she had had a foul, lumpy, green leucorrhea "cured" by local vaginal applications, a few months before. I gave her a dose of *Sepia* (a remedy made from cuttlefish ink) on her mental symptoms. A week later she returned exuberant, all the depression for which she had been doctored being gone, and said, "By the way, doctor, I have that awful discharge back again just as it was before." I was delighted, warned her against suppressing it a second time, and gave *Placebo*. The discharge has since lessened and improved in character and she continues, as her husband says, a changed woman. So much for the fundamental differences.

Another problem which confronted me was whether the homoeopathic remedy could influence definite chronic pathology. A girl of 19 came to me for severe intermenstrual bleeding. On examination I found a nodular fibroid bigger than my fist. A well-known New York specialist, she told me later, had diagnosed it and advised merely general health measures, as he did not want to give X-ray to so young a girl. Her chronic case worked out on mental and general symptoms to *Phosphorus*, which happens to be one of the main remedies useful in fibroids. Three months after I gave her this I sent her to be checked up by the same specialist. He was amazed at the decrease in size of the fibroid and asked her what she had been doing. Six months later he pronounced her normal and sanctioned her marrying.

A further difficulty I experienced was in believing the current statement that homoeopathic remedies can do no harm. THEY CAN!

Another problem which one frequently meets in general practice is that of prophylaxis. Strict homoeopaths believe that vaccines and inoculations are harmful. It took considerable experience for me to be convinced that the chronic constitutional remedy is the

85

best prophylactic. The whole subject of the chronic constitutional remedy is a fascinating one, but beyond the scope of this paper.

As a last problem comes the practical one which is such a stumbling block to students, as to whether one can make a living on homoeopathic general practice. Certainly more than half of my patients were not believers in Homoeopathy, many of them dead against it, but I have found that by up-to-date examination and laboratory procedures, by the actual accomplishment of the remedies, and by adroitly "selling" to the patient the principles of Homoeopathy without the name, they are intrigued, send you their friends, and become staunch believers in the method.

To all of the puzzling problems outlined above, a satisfactory solution can be found, if one is willing to do the hard work involved in learning enough to get results, I am completely "sold" to Homoeopathy. When I fail, I know that the failure is *mine* and not Homoeopathy's and when I can see a similar remedy for a case, I have, even before giving it, a perfect certainty that good results will be forthcoming.

STRANGE, RARE AND PECULIAR SYMPTOMS

A pupil, well along in Homoeopathy, has recently told us that one of his stumbling blocks is the "strange, rare, and peculiar" symptoms. He wants to know what such a symptom is, with examples, whether it may be both a general and a particular, how it affects the evaluation, whether is is equivalent to a keynote, etc.

A "strange, rare, and peculiar" symptom may be of two kinds. It may be a symptom which is weird, fantastic, unheard of, rarely found, such as "sensation in a non-pregnant woman of something alive, jumping about in the abdomen", or "sensation of the whole body being brittle." The second class is that of symptoms which though not fantastic in themselves are unusual, unexpected, and even contrary to what you could rationally predicate in a given condition; for instance, "laughs and sings when in pain"; "thirst for cold during chilly stage only, with no thirst during fever." This latter type, as you will see from the two above examples, is peculiar because of the juxtapositions, it is the concomitance that is queer, "laughter with a pain", thirst with chill."

Such a symptom can be a mental, a general, or a particular; in the nature of things it cannot be a common symptom. As an example of such a mental, take "sensation as if she were double in bed", or "constantly washing the hands"; as a typical strange general take the well known *Camphor* symptom, "desires heat during the hot stages and cold during the cold stages", or "thirsty with aversion to water"; as a rare particular take "empty sensation inside the head", or "blueness of the nails during chill", or "temporary blindness which passes off as the headache develops", or "epistaxis brought on by washing the face in cold water."

A "strange, rare, and peculiar" general, such as "chilly but aggravated from heat", outruns other ordinary generals of the same class, unless there is a general which runs through so many particulars that it is the leading feature of the case; for instance, the case has "suicidal on waking"; "homicidal impulses on waking"; "chilliness only on waking"; "restless when he wakes in the morning." Here it is the aggravation on waking in the morning which is the most marked symptom, and it outranks, for repertorizing purposes, even the mentals, suicidal and homicidal impulses, because these are modifiers of the patient's state on waking rather than his constant condition. Among particular symptoms, also, you give preference to the "strange, rare, and peculiar" ones. Angina pectoris with pain extending up into the occiput would take preference over heart pain extending down the arm, because the former is more strange and unusual. The strange mental symptoms may often be of less value then the peculiar generals or particulars. This is especially true in neurasthenic cases, which often invent and embroider symptoms. In the realm of mentals, especially, we must be sure that a symptom is veridical as we said in a former lecture. Some wise homoeopaths claim that in mental cases it is safer to repertorize by strange and prominent generals and particulars, and to consider the myriad mental symptoms only as part of the general picture, when choosing from the materia medica study of the few remedies that come out highest from the repertory study. As a rule, then, we select the generals and the particulars which are most peculiar, provided always that they are prominent features of the case.

"Strange, rare, and peculiar" symptoms often become keynotes, although not all keynotes are strange symptoms; for instance, "hunger at 11:00 A.M." is a keynote of *Sulphur* but it is not a "strange, rare, and peculiar" symptom; the same with the 4:00-8:00 P.M. aggravation of *Lycopodium;* but a keynote which is also a peculiar symptom is the well-known aggravation from downward motion of *Borax*, or "the more you belch the more you have to belch" of *Ignatia*, or the peculiar symptom which is also a keynote of *Calc.*, *Alum.*, and *Nit. ac.*, "craves indigestible things like chalk, earth, and slate pencils."

The individualization which is so essential a part of Homoeopathy is greatly helped by the understanding and use of "strange, rare, and peculiar" symptoms, which Hahnemann himself especially stressed. It is needless to say that if strange symptoms, found under only a couple of remedies, are permitted to eliminate, they may mislead the student; for instance, we had a case which kept telling us that his twitching was worse during eating and when he sat down at the dining table. This symptom is to be found in the Kent *Repertory* under only one remedy, *Plumbum*, which was not at all the remedy for the whole of this case. These strange symptoms are often difficult to elicit, as patients feel ashamed of telling anything so peculiar, so inconsequential or absurd, yet, especially in simple people, they will crop out, and especially where they are generals they prove of enormous value as *parts* of the totality of the symptoms.

TIMING IN PRESCRIBING

Every good mechanic knows the importance of timing in your car's engine. If the cylinders do not synchronize there is loss of power. In diplomacy timing is of the most vital importance. To philosophers, as well as to athletes, rhythm, which is really timing, is paramount. A beginner in homoeopathic prescribing may take his case magnificently but may have no sense for chronology, for the sequence of cause and effect. Always put dates opposite the illnesses, operations, or catastrophes in the patient's history. After a while you get a sixth sense of how one thing follows another, you see the life of the patient and even of his forebears and progeny as an organic whole. Try to connect the ills to which he is heir with seasons, periodicity, time, meteorological phases. Learn to sense how each little man swings in or out of the master rhythms of the universe.

This same perception of timing applies to the physical examination. It is not sufficient that a man's heart shows no gross organic disturbance on an electrocardiograph; one must, with more senses than we give ourselves credit for, enter into the rhythm of his pulse, his breathing. We must understand the metabolic rhythms of eating, digestion, and elimination, and use such means as will help us determine where the lag is or where the spurt in physiology. We must observe with instruments, with our eyes, ears, noses, and fingers the delicate aberration of human functionings. We must realize how a tiny change in phase or current or magnetic field may have an apparently disproportionate counterpart in health and harmony.

We must somehow pervade the patient with a sense of the necessity of order and rhythm, then we are ready to come to the giving of our healing agent, the similar remedy. An old professor of mine used to say that curing is like peeling an onion, you must begin at the top layer; and it is a sound principle of Homoeopathy that, in an untreated case which requires an acute prescription, the most recent symptoms are the guide to the remedy that you should start with. When you have taken a chronic case from birth on, you should be able to see what remedy this human being needed as an infant, as a child, at puberty, in young adulthood, in maturity and age. At some time in the complete cure of a personality you may, as it were, work back to the basic remedy needed or element lacking many years before, but if you give this substance prematurely you will put your timing off. Only the nosodes can be given with profit, either first or intercurrently, as timing regulators. To borrow a botanical analogy, the nosodes are like the genus and the remedy the species.

The most perilous moment in any homoeopathic cure is that of the second prescription. If you cut in from zeal or panic before your first dose has run its course to the full, you will mix up your case. On the other hand, if you wait too long, you will lose valuable time and may alienate your patient. The expert homoeopath should be able to "smell" when a repetition, change of potency, or another remedy is indicated, and should have the character not to be stampeded or misled by the disease, the patient, the family, the consultant, the nurse, or the family retainers!

Remember your cardinal principles: Never repeat a remedy when the patient himself is improving. Never change a remedy when the symptoms are following Hering's law of cure in the reverse order of the symptoms. Never change your remedy when a discharge or eruption follows the administration.

But there is more to timing than just repetition or change. One can almost include potency selection under timing. The patient's vitality is rhythm and his pathology or suppressions are obstacles. A homoeopathic cure is something of a steeplechase; clock your remedies and your potencies and may the best timing win.

THE VALUE AND RELATION OF DIET TO OUR HOMOEOPATHIC REMEDIES

Homoeopathy is so rich in remedial agents that often its practitioners tend to rely on their drugs alone, and to disregard hygiene and other adjuvants to cure. Especially do they fail to work out diets in detail for their patients. It is essential that they bother to do this for a number of reasons. In the first place, for the "psychological effect" upon the patient. Patients want to feel that every scientific care is being given them, and that the doctor takes flattering pains with them; and they need something to *do*, a call to *active* cooperation on their part. Especially is this last the case when the actual remedy administration is in so pleasant, simple, and sparse a form as Homoeopathy prescribes. In the second place, without any drug of any kind, diet can do wonders for many types of cases, as modern medicine so ably demonstrates.

Let us consider, for instance, the value, without any drug, of strict diets in such diseases as: diabetes, nephritis, high blood pressure, renal colic and the uric acid diathesis, arthritis, gall-stones and jaundice, gastric and duodenal ulcer, mucous colitis, visceroptosis, constipation, obesity, and last, but by no means least, tuberculosis and cancer. Every homoeopathic physician must be grounded in the classical dietary treatments, must know when to give a diabetic the New-burg high fat diet, and the difference between diets for nephritics and nephrotics, must enforce purine-free diets in the chronic renal colics, must be conversant with the Lippe diet for ulcer, and the Lahey-Jordan diet for mucous colitis (with its cream of wheat and celery, whose roughage combined with the concomitant rest prescribed does such wonders in those obstinate cases). The physician must know how to influence acidity, strong urine, asthma, and eczema by dietary means.

It is good training for us, and a helpful method of experimental control of our remedies, to start chronic patients who have some one of the above mentioned diagnoses on diet and regimen plus *Sac. lac.* without any remedy, and see how far we can improve their condition. Thus do we learn what scientific common sense will, and will not, do for us. Meanwhile we are getting closer to the patient's *similimum* and can give it in prepared ground, with startling and enlightening effect.

Diet can often replace the use of drugs—a valuable help for the homoeopath. Take a patient who has been "living" on soda bicarbonate for years. Teach them that soda, chemically alkaline, produces acid, physiologically, in the stomach, and train them to substitute lemon juice and the citrus fruits in general, and watch. You will be amazed that so simple a means will work so well. Meanwhile the soda intoxication symptoms will pass off, and your case values will begin to be unravelled.

The physician must also at the onset remove articles of diet and habits of eating which hold the patient back from cure, and which cover the spoor on the trail to a "totality," and therefore to subsequent healthful progress. He learns on this quest the idiosyncrasies to food on the part of the patient. These, as every homoeopath knows, are of great help and import. In this connection there is a wise rule: *chronic* cases should *not* eat to excess that which they especially crave, whereas *acute* patients *may*—and *should*—eat largely of what they

94

crave, if the craving comes on with the illness. The most extraordinary lapses from classical procedure show admirable results when this rule is followed. *But,* be *sure* that it is a true craving, unusual, individualizing the patient's reaction to the (so-called) acute disease. The cravings for and aversions to food in chronics will, of course, give you sound generals for your hierarchy of symptoms. If, in chronic cases, the remedy is given, it will, little by little, enable the patient to assimilate that food which he craved, and at the same time, quite reasonably, modify the craving. For example, I have an *Argentum nitricum* patient who craved sugar and was ill from it, and who, under *Arg. nit.* no longer craves it, but can eat it with impunity. Similarly, I have a *Calcarea* child who, after *Calc.*, ceased craving chalk and indigestibles, and can assimilate lime from the food. In connection with being made ill by specific articles of food, several interesting points arise: Try at first to see whether it is a combination of foods which disagree, or the one given element of diet. A wise professor once told me that if everyone would drink buttermilk the if they ate it by itself. Next in the case of certain acids, try giving cream or cottage cheese with them. For instance, those with whom strawberries disagree, can often take strawberries if cream cheese is eaten at the same time; similarly with tomatoes. This also applies to shellfish in some patients. Beware the combinations of acids and sugars, starches with meat, in people with delicate digestions. Buttermilk will often so alter the colon's flora and fauna that putrefaction is regulated and much can be digested which hitherto did not agree. A famous German homoeopath, Dr. Schlegel the elder, told me that if everyone whould drink buttermilk the race would profit enormously, and if they would add honey (formic acid) and radishes (which are anti-uric-acid) even more trouble would be saved. Remember that onions help keep blood pressure down (the ex-citable Italians with their garlic and onions rarely have hypertension).

In idiosyncrasies of preference, rather than actual aggravations, ingenuity will save much trouble. Your child or patient who will not take milk may enjoy it if vichy or seltzer be added, or if milk and cream are mixed half and half with ginger ale or sarsaparilla. Or the difference between hot and cold milk may change the dislike.

Those needing iron who claim cabbage gives them gas can often take raw cabbage with sour cream dressing. Spinach pureed with egg chopped on it will tempt the anti-green child. Cider and raw apples are marvelous for thinning the arthritic patient. Brown sugar, molasses, maple syrup, and honey will not harm him as other sweets will. These hints may seem feminine and trivial, but I assure you, they work. I hope the discussion of this paper will prevoke much more lore in this line.

There is another sphere where diet aids materially in cleansing the system. We have mentioned buttermilk and lemon juice. White of egg, with lemon or orange juice, makes a detoxifying liver wash for the bilious. The egg albumen forms albuminates with the poisons which accumulate in the liver. Tea made from red clover blossoms and drunk, two quarts daily, helps the cancer patients and appears to cleanse the system (an old German adjuvant).

So far we have not even mentioned the important relationship between certain foods and the best action of our remedies. But surely you all know these symbioses and antagonisms. For example, *Aconite* and acids do not agree, coffee antidotes the action of *Nux vomica*. These relationships are legion and can be found in Clarke's *Dictionary of Materia Medica* and in many other of our classics, under the separate remedies.

Certain theoretical problems of enormous interest to me come up under this subject. For instance, we use articles of food as remedies. What reaction, if any, may these have on patients sensitive to them, even in the crude, comestible form? And vice versa, can we aid the suitable remedy by giving its crude counterpart as a food simultaneously? Furthermore, should we not make and prove the whole range of vegetables, fruits, and nutritive articles, so that when we find a patient with an idiosyncrasy to something we can compare his case with the proving of the offending food and see whether it may not fit and aid? These foods should be proven on those with a sensitivity to them. For instance, I should prove egg-plant, our friend Dr. Roberts, has proved tomato, and a patient of mine, who is violently ill from even a dash of red pepper lurking in the soup—though he has plenty in his disposition —would make an admirable prover of *Capsicum*.

These last considerations are offered to you as "articles of diet." Think them over, digest them.

THE DANGERS OF HOMOEOPATHIC PRESCRIBING

The greatest danger for any homoeopathic physician is that he will not be a true Hahnemannian homoeopath. Mongrelism defeats not only the doctor and the patient, but also the cause of Homoeopathy. The specific pitfalls most frequently met are as follows:

1. The physician does not bear in mind his homoeopathic philsophy.

2. He fails to take a complete enough case from which to deduce the true remedy. He omits the mentals, the profoundly important generals, or fails to elicit the modalities of the particular symptoms.

3. He lacks patience. Having given the remedy, he forgets that he must WAIT and WATCH. He repeats the remedy in unwise zeal, before the definite slump comes after the improvement which has followed his remedy. More of a good thing does not mean a better thing in homoeopathic prescribing.

4. He fails to look for the action of Hering's three Laws of Cure: That the remedy works *from within outward, from above downward,* and *in the reverse order of the symptoms.* (This never happens except under the action of the curative homoeopathic remedy.)

5. He omits to make use of the "second-best remedy", i.e., *Sac. lac.* Thereby he sometimes loses the

patient's confidence, especially that of those who are accustomed to taking much medicine.

6. He fails to make sure that the patient has actually taken the remedy. (Wherever possible, always administer *the* dose yourself.) Or he fails to find out what other remedies the patient may be taking or what dietetic interferences there are. The physician must be cognisant of what substances interfere with the action of our different remedies, as coffee with *Nux vom.,* or acids with *Acon.*

7. He does not search out the psychological and sociological deterrents to cure and teach the patient how to evade and overcome these.

8. He sometimes does not recognize soon enough when the remedy is *not* working, and is then often too busy to revise the case and try again to find the most similar remedy.

9. He permits himself to give minor remedies for trivial or temporary ailments incident to chronic treatment, when *Sac. lac.* or sensible adjuvants such as hydrotherapy would suffice.

10. He changes the remedy because of the outcropping of other symptoms, without discriminating between aggravation symptoms, symptoms due to idiosyncrasy, symptoms returning under the chronic remedy (which the patient may never recall having had before), actual new symptoms which occur because the remedy was only partially similar, and finally, symptoms of some discharge, such as coryza, leucorrhea, or perspiration, which represent a curative vent and are due to the action of the remedy.

11. He gives the wrong potency of the right remedy. (If sure of the remedy, it is well to try another potency, or first, three doses of the original potency at two or four hour intervals. N.B.: always instruct patients to stop taking the remedy as soon as appreciable amelioration sets in, and to switch to the "second" remedy, i.e., *Sac. lac.*)

12. He gives too high a potency in an incurable case, or in one with marked pathological changes, and so induces an aggravation with which the vital force cannot cope. (If he has done this and the patient is going downhill, he must antidote.)

13. He gives a profound constitutional remedy to a case which is too sick to stand it and which should have merely a related palliative remedy. For instance, in incipient tuberculosis it is dangerous to give *Sulph.*, *Sil.*, or *Phos.*, at least in high potency. A single dose of the thirtieth (30th) is as high as he should venture. If the case is far gone in tuberculosis, these remedies must not be given, but rather a palliative for the most distressing symptoms, such as *Rumex, Sang., Puls.*, or *Seneg.*

14. He must remember that certain remedies are dangerous to mishandle. For instance, *Kali carb.*, especially in cases of advanced arthritis; or *Sil.*, where an abscess, if suppuration were brought on, would break in a dangerous location, as in the lungs; or some of the nosodes, like *Psor.*, which in deeply psoric cases, say of asthma, may induce terrific aggravation; or *Lachesis,* whose *improper repetition may engraft a permanent unfavourable mental state on the patient. Arsenicum* is another dangerous remedy. When apparently indicated in the last stages of an acute disease, say pneumonia, it may hasten demise, although it will make the death tranquil, but it will not rally the patient as one might expect. In the terminal stages of chronic disease, where cure is impossible, it will sometimes bring the patient back long enough to sign a will or see the family, and will ultimately induce euthanasia.

15. He will often be surprised to find that certain symptoms or groups of symptoms are relieved by his remedy and yet the patient feels worse or develops more deeply seated trouble. In this case the prescribing has been superficial and suppressive. Suppression is perhaps the greatest danger of ordinary medicine, from the point of view of homoeopathic philosophy, and the

deep homoeopath must be constantly on his guard not to produce suppression with his remedies. If he has given an acute remedy for an apparently superficial trouble, which is relieved, but the patient feels badly, he should do the chronic case at once, and the deep-acting remedy will right matters.

16. He may give remedies in the wrong order or inimical remedies in succession, thereby aggravating the patient and mixing up the case.

Throughout his practice the physician must sell the idea of Homoeopathy with brief but helpful explanations to the patients, in order to insure their cooperation. He must himself have the character to sit tight when he knows what he is doing, and not spoil his cases by unnecessary and harmful prescribing. Above all, he must consider each patient as an opportunity for service not only to the individual and the community, but to Homoeopathy and to the race.

Elizabeth Wright-Hubbard, M.D.
(18 February 1896-22 May, 1967)

Dr. Wright-Hubbard was one of the foremost homoeopaths of the United States, and in the world. She learned her Homoeopathy from Dr. Pierre Schmidt of Geneva, Switzerland, who had been taught by Dr. A. E. Austin and Dr. F. E. Gladwin, two of Dr. James Tyler Kent's most illustrious pupils. She venerated this great tradition which had formed her, and magnificently served it in her practice and teaching. Her extensive writings are a precious storehouse of homoeopathic knowledge; they will guide and inspire future generations of homoeopathic physicians as they do those of our day. The quintessence of her vast experience and insight has been formulated in this *Brief Course in Homoeopathy*, to which students and masters alike will keep returning, either to learn or to admire.